# The Journey from Student to Paramedic in the UK Ambulance Service

Drawing on extensive ethnographic research, this fascinating book highlights the challenges and contradictions faced by neophyte paramedics as they transition from a classroom setting into day-to-day clinical work placements.

Shining a spotlight on the subculture of the UK Ambulance Service, as well as the paramedic profession more widely, it examines critically how language, cultural meanings, institutionalised rules, professional identity, and working practices determine key behaviours within paramedic practice, providing readers with insight into the profession not seen by members of the public or portrayed by media representations. The book draws on work of seminal authors and experts in the field to provide a sociological perspective on this not only challenging but also, at times, chaotic professional environment.

Supported by fieldnotes as well as interviews with students and paramedics, the book will be essential reading for any student on the path to becoming a paramedic. It will also be valuable reading for those within the service who wish to better understand the hidden cultural and social components that lie beneath the practice itself.

**John Donaghy** is a senior lecturer at Anglia Ruskin University, UK. John has had over 30 years working in an NHS ambulance service, initially as an ambulance man in the late 1970s, prior to becoming a paramedic, first responder, flight paramedic, duty officer, paramedic training officer, and tactical support officer. In addition, he has had over 20 years in academia managing both undergraduate and postgraduate paramedic degree programmes. His research interests lie in the professionalisation of professions.

**Diane Waller** is Emeritus Professor of Art Psychotherapy (Goldsmiths University of London), Hon. President, British Association of Art Therapists, former Council Member (Health and Care Professions Council), and Group Analytic Psychotherapist (UK Council for Psychotherapy). Her research interests include the sociology of health professions, art therapies with people with progressive illness, stroke, and eating disorders, and intercultural therapy. She is also Series Editor (with Sarah Scoble) of Routledge's International Research in the Arts Therapies.

# The Journey from Student to Paramedic in the UK Ambulance Service

Social and Cultural Issues in Paramedic Development

**John Donaghy and Diane Waller**

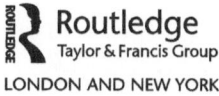

Routledge
Taylor & Francis Group

LONDON AND NEW YORK

Designed cover image: Routledge

First published 2024
by Routledge
4 Park Square, Milton Park, Abingdon, Oxon OX14 4RN

and by Routledge
605 Third Avenue, New York, NY 10158

*Routledge is an imprint of the Taylor & Francis Group, an informa business*

*British Library Cataloguing-in-Publication Data*
A catalogue record for this book is available from the British Library

ISBN: 978-1-032-72141-5 (hbk)
ISBN: 978-1-032-34899-5 (pbk)
ISBN: 978-1-032-72140-8 (ebk)

DOI: 10.4324/9781032721408

Typeset in Sabon
by Apex CoVantage, LLC

# Contents

# About the authors

**Dr John Donaghy (EdD)**, John has had over 30 years employment in an NHS ambulance service, initially as an ambulance person in the late 1970s before undertaking several developmental roles, including paramedic, first responder, flight paramedic, duty officer, paramedic training officer, and tactical support officer. For the past 20 years he has worked in academia, on both undergraduate and postgraduate paramedic degree programmes, initially as a principal lecturer and professional lead/line manager, then as a part-time senior lecturer, which is his current position. His research interests lie in the professionalisation of professions, including the challenging cultures associated with the ambulance service. He is also a member of the Health and Care Professions Council's (HCPC's) fitness to practice (FTP) panel, as well as an HCPC education approval visitor. His clinical work is carried out at Wembley National Stadium.

**Professor Diane Waller (OBE)**, Diane's background is in fine art, ethnography, and group analysis. A Leverhulme European Research Scholarship enabled her to spend a year in Bulgaria and Macedonia, studying the effects of industrialisation on traditional arts. Later she pioneered training in art, group, and intercultural psychotherapy at Goldsmiths and helped to achieve statutory regulation for arts therapies in 1997. She worked extensively in Eastern Europe during the 1980s and 1990s especially Bulgaria and former Yugoslavia, developing new psychosocial services. Her research interests lie in the development of psychotherapies in the United Kingdom and Europe, along with the professionalisation of professions.

# Acknowledgements

We would like to thank our family and friends for the support and encouragement they have given us over this period. Also, we thank all the participants who made this book possible by allowing the research to take place, and we couldn't have done it without you. We would also like to say a special thank you to Routledge for their commitment, understanding, and patience in allowing us to bring this book to fruition.

# Figures

# Tables

# Glossary of terms

| | |
|---|---|
| AACE | Association of Ambulance Chief Executives |
| A&E | Accident and Emergency |
| AFC | Agenda for Change |
| AP | Advanced Practitioner |
| BBC | British Broadcasting Corporation |
| CCP | Critical Care Paramedic |
| COD | Council of Deans for Health |
| COP | College of Paramedics |
| EMT | Emergency Medical Technician |
| GP | General Practitioner |
| HART | Hazardous Area Response Team |
| HCPC | Health and Care Professions Council |
| HEE | Health Education England |
| HEMS | Helicopter Emergency Medical Service |
| HMSO | Her Majesty's Stationary Office |
| ITU | Intensive Care Unit |
| JRCALC | Joint Royal Colleges Ambulance Liaison Committee |
| MAXQDA | Qualitative research supporting software |
| MDT | Mobile Data Terminal |
| NHS | National Health Service |
| NHSTA | National Health Service Ambulance Training Authority |
| NHSTD | National Health Service Ambulance Training Directorate |
| NMC | Nursing Midwifery Council |
| NIHR | National Institute of Health Research |
| NQP | Newley Qualified Paramedic |
| OSCE | Objective Structured Clinical Examination |
| PAD | Practice Assessment Document |
| PPED | Paramedic Practice Educator |
| QAA | Quality Assurance Agency |
| QAP | Qualified Ambulance Person |
| REF | Research Excellence Framework |
| UPR | University Policies and Procedures |

# 1 Introduction

## 1.1 Aims of this book

This book aims to throw light on how and why, following a period of formal university education, undergraduate student paramedics become enculturated, such as how newcomers participate in the normative practices of a cultural group (Kishner & Meng, 2012: 65), into a National Health Service (NHS) ambulance trust.

The book is based around the successful completion of Dr John Donaghy's doctoral thesis following his unique insight into the enculturation of student paramedics' journey into the ambulance workplace. Undertaking an extensive 18-month ethnography, John was able to capture not only the working practices and traditions of the paramedics' workplace but also the intricacies and nuances which underpinned many of these practices. As an experienced paramedic and academic, John was able to position and contextualise much of what he saw and experienced to his work in the ambulance service as he flipped between insider and outsider researcher in the field.

John's findings provide insight into what really goes on in the paramedics and student paramedics workplace. To further strengthen this book, the work introduces these findings to the sociology of workplace practice to try and provide meaning and understanding of these dichotomies. In doing so, Professor Diane Waller (Di), OBE, has provided a rich and meaningful context to the work, as the work draws on Di's extensive knowledge, experience, and understanding of the professionalisation agenda. As an art therapist, Di's work, both nationally and internationally, gives a wider contextualisation of the findings across various disciplines and professions, providing further insight into the book.

For ease of reading, we have therefore used the plural 'we' as we take the reader through each chapter, then the singular 'I', when referring to the ethnographic fieldwork, as John was the principal research investigator. We also use 'I', to highlight Di's personal experiences as she talks about the professionalisation agenda around art therapists.

The book subsequently explores and critically analyses the students' enculturation away from the university to understand the relationship between

DOI: 10.4324/9781032721408-1

two different cultures. The culture which students and neophyte paramedics experience in the clinical practice setting is different from the culture nurtured and experienced by students in university. We ascertain that the culture experienced in the workplace is drawn from the traditional practices and processes embedded within the ambulance service. We suggest that this forms a subculture which subsequently creates a hidden curriculum that students are exposed to. This hidden curriculum gives rise to a form of pedagogy which, in part, inhibits and impedes the students' ability to influence and change the subculture they become accustomed to. To help understand this, an ethnographic approach was adopted to explore, interpret, and illustrate the traditional workplace practices, cultural norms, and hidden curriculum which students, along with neophyte paramedics, experience in the clinical workplace.

## 1.2 Rationale for the book

The rationale for this book followed our initial interest in students returning to university after attending their clinical practice placements. There were distinct differences in the students' behaviours, attitudes, and working practices to that previously seen in the university. We wondered why this was occurring after such a relatively short period of time in clinical practice. In addition, we were aware of the high number of reported fitness to practice (FTP) cases (complaints), being referred to the UK regulator, the Health and Care Professions Council (HCPC, 2023), concerning both experienced and novice paramedics. We were also mindful of the growing number of adverse publications in healthcare, such as the Professional Standards Authority on Managing Poor Performance (2018), Emergency Healthcare in Crisis: Public Services Committee report (2022), and the Kings Fund – An NHS in Crisis: patients are now waiting longer for almost every type of emergency care report (2023). This is in addition to previous high-profile reports like the Francis (2010) report and subsequent Keogh (2013) report, both of which highlighted significant areas of concern, such as poor care, unprofessional behaviours, and poor attitudes which they considered could be widespread.

## 1.3 The research questions

In answering the research question – *The Journey from Student to Paramedic in the UK Ambulance Service: Social and Cultural Issues in Paramedic Development* – several sub-questions emerged, which are listed in the following:

- Why do student paramedics, returning from clinical practice, appear to take on a different form of identity to that previously seen in the university?
- How do student paramedics function in the clinical practice-based environment?
- How do students contextualise their academic studies into real-life practice-based situations and experiences?

- What are the working relationships between the students and their colleagues (crewmates)?
- What are the working relationships between the students and managers?
- What are the working relationships between the students and patients/ public and wider healthcare community?
- What is the changing agency of a specific form of learning, which may shape the students' ways of working?

These were all questions which we needed to understand. To fulfil these objectives, ethnography provided a suitable research approach. Subsequently, as the paramedic, I (John) would observe a group of university student paramedics over an intense period of 18 months as they attended their day-to-day clinical work placements. This allowed me to witness the students' real-life experiences, along with the intricacies and nuances of their day-to-day work. As in the research, observational fieldnotes were used, along with audio recordings and recorded reflective and reflexive notes to capture the day-to-day practices of both the students and experienced paramedics. I was able to reflect on my observations and clarify the fieldnotes with follow-up interviews and conversations with the students and paramedics. Riemann (2012) suggests the written work is a synthesis of the researcher's impressions which are recorded as fieldnotes, observations, or interview data. In collecting the fieldnotes, several issues arose from the data. For example, students mimicked their paramedic colleagues' behaviours and attitudes, they made derogatory comments about patients, and, at times, students were coerced into avoiding emergency calls along with occasionally damaging ambulances, such as kicking and damaging the dashboard. These issues are explored in more detail in the proceeding chapters. From the fieldwork, we found that students internalise and interpret the placement setting differently to that previously taught in university, which further adds to the dichotomies experienced by students. How they are influenced by and interact with the traditional cultures of the workplace and their perception of themselves within the paramedic environment are explored. We needed to understand the various cultural meanings which students came to interpret as normal practice, such as those identified by Devenish et al. (2016), Becker et al. (1961), and O'Meara (2011), as these are essential components of the socialisation process. At times throughout the book, we use the terms enculturation and socialisation interchangeably. However, it is important that we define the two terms and their respective differences at the outset. Therefore, we very simply define these terms as follows: socialisation is a process of learning to behave in a way that is acceptable to society, whereas enculturation is the process of being socialised in a certain culture.

Within the research we argue that students, when on placement, are drawn into a different form of practice. This form of practice influences and impedes the pedagogy to that experienced in the university. The early work of Metz (1981) goes some way in supporting this, suggesting it is because of the traditions and practices embedded within the very fabric of the ambulance service workplace that these practices occur.

## 1.4  Structure of the book

In Chapter 2, the description of the recent history of the NHS ambulance service and paramedic profession is laid out. Some of the traditional processes and events which have influenced and impacted on the development of the ambulance service and paramedic profession are identified. By doing this, a degree of insight and understanding into the ambulance service helps contextualise the traditional working practices and customs associated with the UK ambulance service. The degree to which these traditions have become an integral and inseparable part of the ambulance service gives rise to the very essence of enculturation. We reflect on our own knowledge, to help identify key milestones in the development of the ambulance service and paramedic profession, both as experienced paramedic and educationalist and art therapist and educationalist/researcher (Di Waller), who was instrumental in establishing regulation of art therapy as part of their professionalisation agenda which began in the early 1960s with the formation of the British Association of Art Therapists (BAAT). Key milestones are identified in the development of the paramedic profession. Lastly, a reflexive stance is used to help position these developments within today's practices.

In Chapter 3, we explore the literature. The culture, the subculture, and the hidden curriculum associated with student paramedics' enculturation are reviewed and interrogated. This helps identify and understand the resulting pedagogy. The stringent organisational structures of the NHS ambulance service, to that of the day-to-day work of student paramedics and experienced paramedics, are further explored to possibly help identify the two competing cultures, which Schein's (1985) model of organisational culture helps to illustrate. The notion of professionalisation and the professional identity of paramedics are examined as we illustrate how paramedic storytelling becomes an integral part of the day-to-day narrative of paramedics and student paramedics. Finally, Lave and Wenger's (1991) work on Communities of Practice is explored to help bring the work together to provide meaning and understanding of how and why students become enculturated into the organisation.

In Chapter 4, the methodology and the research processes are identified. We discuss how a constructivist paradigm was used in the research and how ethnography became the primary methodology for the study. The research methods used to obtain the data are identified to help reveal the students' experiences, as Becker et al. (1961: 133) believe, 'the most complete form of sociological datum, after all, is the form in which the participant observer gathers it, this rich data gives more information about the event under study, than data gathered by any other sociological method'. Where the research was conducted, along with the details of the participants and the duration of the study, is discussed. Lastly, the thematic analyses and management of the data were carried out, along with the supporting software which helped us to review and revise various themes and trends emerging from the initial analysis of the data.

Chapter 5 provides a comprehensive look at the research findings. The challenges and opportunities of riding out in the ambulance with students and experienced paramedics are illuminated. A key theme drawn from the data revolves around the work experiences of students, neophyte paramedics, and experienced paramedics. Tensions developed in the clinical practice setting between crew staff, students, and mentors, with managers and at times with patients and the public. Issues such as harassment and bullying are further drawn out of the fieldnotes and represented in the narrative of the findings. The institutionalisation of the ambulance service and its relationship to the paramedics' working environment are discussed, as these also became key themes which emerged from the data. Finally, the relationship of dark (black) humour, which Scott (2007) suggests is an essential component of the paramedics' day-to-day work, is discussed.

In Chapter 6, we discuss how the three dominant constructs, work experience, professional identity, and organisational culture, are woven throughout the narrative of the work. We show that the findings reveal forms of student enculturation which influences and impacts upon the student learning. We argue that the pedagogy emerging from the practice placement experience is not reflective of the pedagogy which students experience in the university classroom setting.

In Chapter 7, we look at the implications for practice and put forward some recommendations for long-term change. We reflect on our work as we unravel the initial research question to summarise the basis of the study. We highlight the strengths and limitations of the study. Finally, apart from McCann's (2022) excellent publication, there is limited recent published literature around the socialisation of student paramedics into the UK ambulance service. Much of the published literature focuses on patient care and clinical presentations, diagnosis, and treatment. The book concludes by depicting how the study adds to the limited published research on the workplace socialisation of student paramedics in the UK.

This chapter provides an outline of the research. The next chapter provides a historical overview of the developments of the paramedic profession over the past 40 years.

## References

Becker, H., Geer, B., Hughes, C. E. & Strauss, L. A. (1961) *Boys in White*. New Brunswick, NJ: Transaction Books.

Devenish, A. S., Clark, M. J. & Fleming, M. L. (2016) *Experience in Becoming a Paramedic: The Professionalisation of University Qualified Paramedics*. Brisbane, Australia: Faculty of Health, Queensland University of Technology.

Emergency Healthcare – A National Emergency. (2022) https://committees.parliament.uk/publications/33569/documents/187215/default/

Francis, R. (2010) *Independent Inquiry into Care Provided by Mid Stafford NHS Foundation Trust January 2005 – March 2009*. London: The Stationery Office.

Health and Care Professions Council. (2023) https://www.hcpc-uk.org/

Keogh, B. (2013) *Review into the Quality of Care and Treatment Provided by 14 Hospital Trusts in England: Overview Report*. London: National Health Service.

Kings Fund. (2023) https://www.kingsfund.org.uk/blog/2023/01/nhs-crisis-patients-now-waiting-longer-every-type-emergency-care

Kishner, D. & Meng, L. (2012) *Enculturation and Acculturation: Encyclopaedia of the Sciences of Learning*. Boston, MA: Springer.

Lave, J. & Wenger, E. (1991) *Situated Learning: Legitimate Peripheral Participation*. Cambridge: Cambridge University Press.

McCann, L. (2022) *The Paramedic at Work – A Sociology of a New Profession*. Oxford: Oxford University Press.

Metz, L. D. (1981) *Running Hot-Structure and Stress in Ambulance Work*, 1st ed. Edited by L. D. Metz. Cambridge, MA: Abt Books.

O'Meara, P. (2011) 'So how can we frame our identity?', *Journal of Paramedic Practice*. paramedicpractice.com.

Professional Standards Authority. (2018) https://www.professionalstandards.org.uk/docs/default-source/conferences/presentation/2018-conference/weenink.pdf?sfvrsn=fada7220_2

Riemann, G. (2012) 'Self-reflective ethnographies of practice and their relevance for professional socialisation in social work', *International Journal of Action Research*, 7(3), pp. 262–293.

Schein, H. E. (1985) *Organisational Culture and Leadership*, 2nd ed. San Francisco, CA: Jossey-Bay.

Scott, T. (2007) 'Expression of humour by emergency personnel involved in sudden death work', *Mortality*, 12(4), pp. 350–364.

# 2  Historical context

## 2.1 Introduction

In this section of the book, several key events are identified, which have shaped and influenced today's representation of the modern-day NHS ambulance service. The work of Case et al. (2014) believes ethnography provides a historical, deeply contextual, and in-depth understanding of communities, which is used in this study. We briefly explore the past, to shed light on the future role of the paramedic.

To help understand student paramedics' enculturation into the ambulance service, this overview of historical content helps contextualise the paramedic journey over the past 40+ years. We illustrate how the embryonic nature of paramedic development provides insight into the rapid growth of knowledge which paramedics are now expected to obtain, in terms of psychomotor practical skills, such as inserting a cannula (needle) into a patient's vein and correctly maintaining a patent airway on unconscious patients who have a suspected spinal injury, along with the cognitive clinical knowledge and application of care, such as anatomy and physiology, pathophysiology, and pharmacology. Highlighting the trajectory of the ambulance service, along with the development of the paramedic profession over this period, provides a historical overview in which to distinguish between the traditional working conditions and practices of the 1970s and that of the modern-day (2023) NHS ambulance service and paramedic profession.

## 2.2  The Millar report

We start with a summary of the National Health Service Act (1946), which called for local authorities to provide ambulances, as and when necessary, to the public. This provided a basic system of transportation for the sick or injured to hospital. This basic form of transportation remained for many years against a backdrop of post-war austerity and deprivation. In 1966, in the midst of seeking improved pre-hospital care, Dr E Millar reported to the minister of health on the standard of equipment and training requirements for the NHS ambulance staff. The report, known as the Millar report (Millar,

DOI: 10.4324/9781032721408-2

1966), became instrumental in enhancing the standards of training for ambulance crews. However, this training mainly consisted of psychomotor skills to help aid the introduction of new pieces of ambulance equipment, such as splints, oxygen, and dressings, along with some limited technology, such as radios. The Millar standard remained as a recognised component of ambulance training for several years, only to be superseded in the 1980s by the introduction of the National Health Service Ambulance Training Authority (NHSTA), later to become the National Health Service Ambulance Training Directorate (NHSTD). The NHSTD standardised training (Kilner, 2004) and provided the syllabus for advanced ambulance training into the 1980/1990s, although this did not completely replace Millar, rather complemented the Millar standard.

## 2.3  Cultural boundaries

To help provide an indication of the level of trained ambulance staff of the 1970s and illustrate the cultural community in which staff worked at that time, we draw on the work of Morris (1970), who provides a sense of the workforce in his work on the role of the ambulance woman:

> Female ambulance attendants are employed by some ambulance Authorities, but obviously the duties which they can perform normally have to be of a limited nature. Their true value comes in the daily transportation of the more mobile out-patients, using the sitting-car type vehicle, and in dealing with old people and children.
>
> I would not in any way decry the worth of female ambulance attendants, because they do most certainly ease the out-patient workload, allowing more double (male) crews to be available for emergency work.
>
> The female ambulance attendant would be advised to undergo a period of training similar to that of her male counterpart, especially, comprehensive first aid, kinetics, the handling of the elderly, and good roadcraft. But perhaps some special emphasis might be placed on more sedentary aspects of the service, i.e., work in Control, preparation of work etc., in case relief should be required in that department.
>
> (Morris, 1970)

The discrepancy between male and female workers, along with their expected roles and limitations within the ambulance service, is clear to see and provides an indicator of the culture of that time. Current data depicts a very different picture, suggesting the total number of registered paramedics in 2018/2019 was 27,747 of which 16,916 were males and 10,916 were females and 1 unknown (HCPC, 2022). It should be acknowledged that current trends in gender alignment may depict a different picture today, as non-binary and other gender alignments are recognised and acknowledged in today's society. From the current data, it is reasonable to assume that the culture of the present-day ambulance service should therefore be very different from that of the 1970s.

## 2.4 The Institute of Health Care and Development awards

By the 1980s, as part of the Institute of Health Care and Development (IHCD), technician and paramedic-training award, a national standard for ambulance/paramedic training was mirrored across much of the UK. The curricula, however, predominantly focused on the anatomy and physiology of three predominant systems, namely the respiratory, cardiovascular, and neurological systems of the body, with little context to other anatomical body systems. The curricula were limited in terms of theoretical content in areas such as professional behaviours, healthcare economy, communication strategies, law and ethics, continuous professional development (CPD), reflective practice, and so on. It was, to all intents and purposes, an in-house skills-based approach to advanced training (Brooks et al., 2015). In 1998, an influential report, *Life in the Fast Lane* (The National Audit Office, 1998), highlighted several recommendations for the UK ambulance services, regarding vehicles, patient treatment, equipment, and, more importantly, targets, such as response times.

## 2.5 National ambulance service dispute

In the latter part of 1980, negotiations commenced between ambulance workers and employers. The aim was to agree a national formula which would ensure improved pay and working conditions, such as additional annual leave, negotiated shift rosters, and general improvements in the working terms and conditions of ambulance workers. The collapse of lengthy negotiations between various unions, including the National Union of Public Employees (NUPE), the National Union of General Municipal Workers (NUGMW), the Confederation of Health Service Employees (COHSE), and the then Secretary of State for Health, the Right Honourable Kenneth Clarke MP, led to a nationwide ambulance service dispute.

The dispute became a bitter and difficult fight between the Conservative Government of Margaret Thatcher and the unions which lasted for six months from September 1989 to February 1990. It could now be argued however that due to the dispute, substantial changes emerged in relation to the development of ambulance staff which paved the way in shaping the future direction of the ambulance service, to that of today's ambulance/paramedic provision. The dispute eventually ended in a perceived victory by 'driving a coach and horses through the Government's pay policy' (Poole, 1990: 3). This victory was however contested by many ambulance workers who considered they had been let down by their union representatives. However, I

(John) can recall from my time on the picket line throughout the dispute that the camaraderie of staff was exceptional. Because of the dispute, pay and conditions improved for staff, whilst the creation of the Joint Royal Colleges Ambulance Liaison Committee (JRCALC) provided both clinical guidance and advice to ambulance services. Made up of various medical experts and specialists in pre-hospital emergency care, the group established a set of clinical procedures and governance standards to support ambulance staff in their day-to-day work. These guidelines became known as the National Clinical Guidelines (NCG) and are still used today by the UK paramedics. The NCG provide paramedics with a set of clinical procedures to follow, such as drug doses, clinical algorithms, and clinical advice, which can be referred to in supporting clinical decision making. The JRCALC, along with the then, newly formed professional body, the British Paramedic Association (BPA), provided a national platform of support and guidance to the UK ambulance services.

**(More about this period can be found in Leo McCann's *The Paramedic at Work: A Sociology of a New Profession*: Oxford University Press, 2022, pp. 1–29). This invaluable book was published after this research was completed.)

## 2.6 The move to higher education

Before we examine any impact higher education may have had on paramedic development, we outline how paramedics initially became registered with the Council for Professions Supplementary to Medicine (CPSM) in 1998, along with Clinical Scientists and Speech and Language Therapists. These three disciplines made up the last of the 12 professions allowed to be regulated under the CPSM Act of 1961. The first paramedic university programme began in 1996 and the Paramedic Board only formed just before the Health Act of 2000, which replaced the CPSM and created the Health Professions Council (HPC) – a multi-professional regulator. As most of the other CPSM professions had been regulated since 1961 and had developed university degree programmes which already had strong professional bodies supporting them, paramedics were in a vulnerable place having to get used to being regulated so quickly when they had barely formed any form of professional identity. This is relevant for the argument in this book around professional identity and professionalism, which is why we illustrate this at this juncture in the book. The status of 'emerging profession' was shared by arts therapists (Art, Drama, and Music Therapists) who had combined their resources as professional bodies in order to petition for statutory regulation with the CPSM. The CPSM was undergoing massive changes and so were the professions they regulated in that they were moving away from training in the NHS schools into the higher education sector. The effects of the European Directives were obvious, together with the potential for repealing the old Act and bringing in a new one, more suited to the 1990s than the 1940s and 1950s post-Second World War society. Having met the criteria for a 'new profession' and gained approval from the CPSM, along with Prosthetists and Orthotists, Art Therapists were waiting for the department of health approval to proceed to legislation. Di was attending the CPSM as an 'observer' and remembers how surprised members were at the rapid introduction of Clinical Scientists, Speech and Language Therapists and Paramedics to the group waiting approval. Di recalls:

> We were really taken aback by this development. We knew that the new Bill that would create the Health Professions Council would radically change the way that the professions were regulated. We were aware that there were 3 more places in the CPSM yet to be filled. There was usually a lengthy process of moving from CPSM's approval of a new profession to having that approval ratified by the DOH then moving to an amendment of the CPSM Act to register a new profession. Indeed, it was proving so for Arts Therapists. There seemed to be a distinct reluctance from the Department of Health to recognise that the Arts Therapies should be regulated and this was because of a longstanding lack of understanding of our role, indeed of our value in health care. I remember one meeting at Hannibal House (DoH headquarters then) when one civil servant asked: 'Why do music therapists need regulation just for playing records of Beethoven?' To be fair, he later owned up to being 'mortified' when he learned what their job actually entailed! Later, another official declared that lengthening art therapy training from one year to two years postgraduate was 'spectacularly ill-timed and inflationary. As representatives of our professional bodies, we engaged in a major exercise seeking support across the UK from the hundreds of employers of arts therapists, senior medical and academic colleagues and patients, citing research and publications that clearly explained the level of the profession and the risk of not regulating. When the real substance of our role was at last understood, it was evident that damage could be (and indeed had been) done by unregulated persons misusing our titles. These written statements were delivered to the Department much to the astonishment of the civil servant in charge of our case! In addition, a thorough costing of such a lengthening of training to the NHS was found to be around £10,000 with the costs of this training being mainly born by students of art therapy! Not long after this episode, we were given the Green Light to proceed. While waiting for the DoH to make up its mind, myself and my dramatherapist colleague were able to observe the final stages of the CPSM, the passing of the Health Professions Bill and the moves towards the new Council. We understood that to use the 12 places available on CPSM, three more professions that met their approval criteria could be put forward. That one of these was the Paramedics was somewhat surprising given that there was no professional body then, and that the training differed so radically from that of the other professions. All

these had moved towards undergraduate or even postgraduate education and were seeking much more autonomy than before. The term "Supplementary to Medicine" had long been an irritant and deemed out of date, a feature of the old CPSM Act of 1961 and not reflective of modern working practice and status (female practitioners sometimes being referred to as "handmaidens"!). There was a lot of concern about status and to be honest, not much understanding about the role of paramedics. However, I remember thinking that they were having similar struggles to Arts Therapists in developing their profession, even though Arts Therapies development had been based in universities since the 1970s and was at a postgraduate level. The fact that paramedics had already moved towards a university based training and the extent of their actual contribution, was not known to most of us on the CPSM Council and almost certainly not to the general public. Our struggles were of a different nature but none the less a major challenge in terms of perception and being taken seriously as a profession. The notion of profession as an "honorary symbol" or as a signifier of "knowledge and power" (Johnson, T: Professions and Power (1972) was still strong at that time.' Recently, reflecting on this period, I wondered if the relative ease of enculturation of arts therapy students into the NHS might have been because arts therapists felt strong ownership of the profession, having battled together on many occasions to reach an agreed point. All major decisions had been passed at professional body AGMs from the 1970s onwards. There was little sense of 'old timers' versus newly qualified although obviously some concerns were voiced by those who had been working in the NHS prior to postgraduate training. Grandparenting via the professional bodies seemed to allay these concerns.

The shift in paramedic development into higher education became the catalyst of the gradual decline of the traditional model of in-house training, provided by ambulance services and other external agencies. Considering this, the number of universities developing paramedic diploma programmes, foundation degree programmes, and honours degree programmes increased substantially. The shift in paramedic development into universities spanned several years and faced a degree of strong opposition from several stakeholders, some of which were trade unions, some ambulance crew staff, and a number of ambulance chief officers. Without the continuous drive from organisations such as the BPA, now the College of Paramedics (COP), along with prominent individuals within the paramedic and ambulance sector, such as Furber, Newton, Woolard, Williams, Hunt, Dean, Fellows, Whitmore, and Donaghy, to name a few, in helping to secure the transition into higher education, the transition and direction of paramedic development could have taken a different course.

Having established the transition of paramedic development into higher education and following a public consultation in 2018, the education threshold entry level for paramedics onto the HCPC register was raised from a certificate of higher education or equivalent, to degree-level education. This meant that paramedic programmes, which were still being carried out 'in-house' by ambulance services or other external agencies, may no longer be valid after September 2021. Considering this, existing paramedic programmes, which were delivered below the new threshold degree as entry-level qualification in universities, would no longer be available. Existing paramedics working without a degree-level qualification, but registered on the HCPC register, had the right to continue operating as usual under the auspices of 'grandparenting rights'. The regulatory term used to allow those paramedics registered through previous educational routes to continue to practise as paramedics.

## 2.7 Influential policy documents

In this section various government policies and reports which have impacted and contributed to the working environment of paramedics are examined. These reports depict and imply both the role and scope of paramedic practice, paramedic development, and the role of the paramedic in an evolving NHS. We provide this to give a sense of how these reports continue to contribute and influence the working environment of paramedics and student paramedics. In addition, several key reports are identified as pivotal documents – such as 'Taking healthcare to the patient' – which advocated a model of pre-hospital care involving patients being treated more effectively within their home environment, avoiding unnecessary admission to hospital (Bradley, 2005). This influential report supports the need for an all-graduate profession, suggesting this would adequately equip paramedic students with the necessary knowledge, skills, and attributes required to make accurate informed autonomous clinical diagnostic and management decisions. Darzi's (2008) report inevitably supports an all-graduate pathway by outlining a vision of care which is both accessible and acceptable to patients. This would allow a standardised level of care, regardless of demographics. Newton (2012) provides evidence of the strong research base which is contributing to a higher level of education within the profession, as it equips the paramedics with enhanced knowledge and skills to perform their role. Despite this, the report entitled Paramedic Evidence Based Education Project (Lovegrove, 2013) found models of paramedic education within the UK paramedic profession somewhat diverse, at times lacking structure and continuity in some areas. Similar observations were also made by the Commission on Human Medicines (2015). These publications are important as they are, in part, responsible for the development of paramedic practice (Donaghy, 2008; Cooper, 2005; Woollard, 2006) often set against a position of fiscal austerity across all public sector funding streams (Stevens, 2004), along with an uncertain political landscape (Valderas et al., 2009). National policy documents inevitably influence working practices by establishing targets and creating standards, for example time targets, quality control standards, clinical governance, and so on.

As a result of the aforementioned discussion, Kilner's (2004) Delphi study illustrates how various attributes which experts regarded sufficient for a range of ambulance personnel, including emergency medical technicians (EMTs), paramedics, and supervisors (mentors), inform and question paramedic development. Kilner's (2004) study drew on a panel of experts with specific knowledge of the demands of contemporary pre-hospital emergency care, including ambulance medical directors, members of the JRCALC, the Royal College of Surgeons of Edinburgh, and various advisors to the NHS ambulance service trusts. The study categorised 25 broad statements elicited from 3,403 initial responses to individual statements. The results revealed that many of the desirable areas of learning identified within the study were not embedded within the traditional training curriculum at that time. Areas such as reflective practice, ethics and law, advanced practice, enhanced skills, communication skills, inter-professional working, human factors, resilience, and research were absent from the curriculum. These results indicate that the basic model of in-house training proposed by Millar was predominantly a skill-orientated model, 'as is its modern manifestation of Ambulance Basic and Paramedic training, which places emphasis on technical skills procedures' (Kilner, 2004: 374). The results of the study helped bring the original paramedic training paradigm, consisting of elements of the original IHCD training award, to an end.

These stringent formal policies and rules, which contribute to advancing clinical practice, can also create barriers to autonomous practice by restricting, restraining, and impeding practice. McCann et al. (2015) imply that some of these policies and reports lead to stringent and often unrealistic demands and targets being placed on the workforce. Bradley (2005) lays out the relationship between the expected delivery of ambulance services and the actual delivery of service. The report claims practitioners must obtain additional diagnostic and clinical reasoning skills enabling greater autonomy for paramedics and subsequently improved care pathways for patients. Although, establishing a system whereby healthcare professionals, such as paramedics explore different care options, for example, leaving patients at home if it is safe to do so, contacting social services for patient support instead of leaving vulnerable patients at home, making arrangements for a general practitioner (GP) to attend the patient or some other form of care rather than attending the accident and emergency (A&E) department, are versions of alternative care pathways. In contrast, these alternative care pathways are often perceived by ambulance crews as wholly inadequate since many of these pathways are not necessarily available to the healthcare practitioner or patient. This can cause frustration, anxiety, and sometimes tension amongst paramedic practitioners and graduating paramedic students, as the lack of access to these facilities can lead to a rigid adherence to more traditional ways of working, such as taking all patients to hospital as opposed to using alternative care pathways thus avoiding treatment options and advanced clinical care. We argue this then has the potential to restrict and dictate the healthcare landscape, rather than supporting autonomous clinical practice proposed by the College of Paramedics (2015) and supported by Health Education England (2013).

## 2.8 Today's healthcare professional

The notion of professionalisation of the paramedic profession remains an embryonic development. Bledsoe et al. (2005) consider certain qualities are needed by the practitioner to be a professional, offering the notion that paramedics fall within this, as they contribute to the continuum of care and therefore possess certain qualities to undertake this role, suggesting that the practitioner should be:

> A confident leader who faces up to challenges, accepts responsibility, have excellent judgment skills, be able to prioritise decisions, act quickly in the interest of the patient/client, develop a rapport with a wide variety of people, communicate with diverse cultural groups and ages, be an evidence-based autonomous practitioner.
>
> (Bledsoe et al., 2005: 35)

To fulfil the requirements of professional registration paramedics are expected to underpin their day-to-day practice by adhering to professional standards, such as those prescribed by the HCPC's Standards of Proficiency for Paramedics (2023) and Standards of Conduct, Performance and Ethics (2016). However, as also seen in the work of van der Gaag and Donaghy (2013), these concepts are not always fully understood by some paramedics, as we further argue that the notion of paramedic professionalisation is still unclear and undefined, which is discussed in more detail in Chapter 6.

## 2.9 Professional body

The introduction of the professional body, the COP, provides direction in moving the profession to the next stage of its development (Cooper, 2005), offering professional guidance and opportunities for paramedics to help maintain and enhance individuals' professional profiles. For example, CPD, conferences, outstanding achievement awards, and presentations. The then chair of the COP stated:

> Perhaps the single biggest prize that we still need to seize, is unlocking the full potential of our profession and this means making paramedics ever more relevant and effective in meeting emerging patient needs, through the development of scope of practice.
>
> (Newton, 2011: 58)

Whilst collecting the data, we found there was often confusion and misunderstanding from both students and paramedics as to the role and nature of the various professional, regulatory, advisory, mandatory, and statutory bodies. An example of this is given later to illustrate the various organisations involved in the development and management of the UK ambulance service and paramedic profession: the Ambulance Service Association (ASA) – now the Association of Ambulance Chief Executives (AACE), the IHCD, the JRCALC, the HCPC, the COP, Health Education England (HEE), the Council of Deans for Health (COD), along with various trade unions. These organisations all have different functions and activities which were often unclear, confusing, and not deemed to be important for many students, neophyte, and experienced paramedics.

### 2.9.1 Summary

Over the past 40+ years the development of paramedics has seen a substantial shift from the IHCD training award, predominantly delivered in-house by local and regional ambulance training centres, towards an academic award.

This change of delivery is in keeping with the professional body, the COP, Curriculum Guidance Framework (COP, 2019), which acts as an educational basis for future paramedic education. However, this framework is not isolated and is therefore shaped by the HCPC's Standards of Proficiency for Paramedics (2023), Standards of Education and Training (2017), Standards of Conduct, Performance and Ethics (2016), and the Quality Assurance Agency (QAA) Benchmark Statements (2019). Collectively these organisations support and enhance both paramedic education and the future development of the profession through rigorous frameworks. As Donaghy (2008: 31) suggests, 'these frameworks represent new ways of working for paramedics as front-line practitioners'.

The professional body, along with stakeholders such as the UK Department of Health and Social Care (DHSC), endorses the current shift from a traditional training paradigm, to one of higher education. The move implies students will graduate with a higher degree of knowledge, skills, and professional accountability (Woollard 2009), which will enhance the profession, along with patient care (Donaghy, 2010). As universities continue to establish paramedic programmes to meet the educational needs of the paramedic profession, it is unclear how this will impact on the national shortage of paramedics, which appears to increase exponentially year on year, see NHS Employers (2018). The chaotic and relentless ebb and flow of paramedics moving across from the public sector into the private sector and other healthcare settings, such as private ambulance organisations, private healthcare clinics, industry, accident and emergency (A&E) departments, sporting and leisure facilities, and general practitioner (GP) surgeries, is unprecedented in the UK ambulance services.

We hope this chapter has provided a brief insight into the ambulance/paramedic development over the past 40+ years. Key events and milestones in the development have been alluded to and contextualised within the paramedic journey. The relationship between indicative policies and current paramedic professional development has been discussed, although it could be argued that some of the key influential reports run counter to the autonomy and degree of clinical decision making expected of the modern practitioner, see Lovegrove (2013) and Newton (2012). In this summary, insight into the training and culture associated with the ambulance service of the 1970s have been identified to that expected of today's paramedics. The next chapter explores the literature underpinning this research.

## References

Bledsoe, E. B., Porter, S. R. & Cherry, A. R. C. (2005) *Essentials of Paramedic Care*. Toronto, ON: Brady, p. 35.

Bradley, P. (2005) *Taking Healthcare to the Patient*. Department of Health. DH Publications Orderline. https://ircp.info/Portals/11/Future/NHS%20EMS%20Policy%20Recommendation2005.pdf

Brooks, I. A., Cook, M., Spencer, C. & Archer, F. (2015) 'A review of key national reports to describe the development of paramedic education in England (1966–2014)', *Prehospital Care Emergency Medical Journal*, 33, pp. 876–881.

Case, A. D., Tobb, N. R. & Kral, M. J. (2014) 'Ethnography in community psychology: Promises and tensions', *American Journal of Community Psychology*, (54), pp. 60–71. https://doi.org/10.1007/s10464-014-9648-0

College of Paramedics – Curriculum Guidance. (2015) https://nasemso.org/wp-content/uploads/UKParamedic_Curriculum_Guidance_2015.pdf

College of Paramedic's Curriculum Guidance Framework. (2019) https://collegeof paramedics.co.uk/?gclid=Cj0KCQjwqs6lBhCxARIsAG8YcDhZ5NQeSilXkhny3r CZar2RjVxkoY--4ecNyLV8wg-3THvxjpoD0R0aAqrfEALw_wcB

Commission on Human Medicines – Paramedic Prescribing. (2015) https://pharmaceutical-journal.com/article/news/independent-prescribing-by-paramedics-under-consideration

Cooper, S. (2005) 'Contemporary UK paramedic training and education. How do we train? How should we educate?', *Emergency Medical Journal*, 22, pp. 375–379.

Council for Professions Supplementary to Medicine. (1961) https://www.legislation.gov.uk/ukpga/Eliz2/8-9/66/crossheading/establishment-of-a-council-and-boards-for-certain-professions-supplementary-to-medicine/enacted

Darzi, A. (2008) *Framework for Action, High Quality Care for All*. London. http://www.healthcareforlondon.nhs.uk

Donaghy, J. (2008) 'Higher education for paramedics – Why?', *Journal of Paramedic Practice*, 1, pp. 31–35.

Donaghy, J. (2010) 'Equipping the student for the workplace changes in paramedic education', *Journal of Paramedic Practice*, 2(11), pp. 524–528.

Health Education England. (2013) *Delivering High Quality, Effective, Compassionate Care: Developing the Right People with the Right Skills and the Right Values*. A mandate from the Government to Health Education England: April 2013 to March 2015. London: Department of Health.

Johnson, T. (1972) *Professions and Power*. London: Macmillan.

HCPC Standards of Conduct, Performance and Ethics, London. (2016) London. https://www.hcpc-uk.org/resources/standards/standards-of-conduct-performance-and-ethics/

HCPC Standards of Education and Training. (2017) London. https://www.hcpc-uk. org/resources/guidance/standards-of-education-and-training-guidance/

Health and Care Professions Council. (2022) London. https://www.hcpc-uk.org/

Health and Care Professions Council. (2023) London. https://www.hcpc-uk.org/ standards/standards-of-proficiency/

Kilner, T. (2004) 'Desirable attributes of the ambulance technician, paramedic, and clinical supervisors', *Emergency Medical Journal*, 21, pp. 374–378.

Lovegrove, M. (2013) *Paramedic Evidence Based Education Project (PEEP): Maximising Paramedic' Contribution to the Delivery of High Quality and Cost-Effective Patient Care.* Buckinghamshire: Bucks New University, Allied Health Solutions.

McCann, L., Granter, E., Hassard, J. & Hyde, P. (2015) ' "You can't do both – Something will give": Limitations of the targets culture in managing UK health care workforces', *Human Resource Management*, 54(5), pp. 773–791.

Millar Report. (1966) *Independent Ambulance Service Regulation.* London: Life in the Fast Lane. Audit Commission for Local Authorities and the National Health Service in England and Wales. Audit Commission. ISBN-13 978-1862400641.

Morris, S. (1970) *A Complete Handbook for Professional Ambulance Personnel.* Birmingham: Wright.

National Audit Commission. (1998) *Life in the Fast Lane: Value for Money in Emergency Ambulance Services.* London. https://www.nao.org.uk/wp-content/ uploads/2017/01/NHS-Ambulance-Services.pdf

National Health Service Act. (1948) https://www.parliament.uk/about/living-heritage/ transformingsociety/livinglearning/coll-9-health1/health-01/

National Health Service Employers. (2018) https://www.nhsemployers.org/articles/ framework-agreement-2018-pay-deal

Newton, A. (2011) 'Specialist practice for paramedics: A bright future', *Journal of Paramedic Practice*, 3(2).

Newton, A. (2012) 'The ambulance service: The past, present and future (part 1)', *Journal of Paramedic Practice*, 4(5), p. 8.

Poole, R. (1990) Cited in Steel, P. (2015) 'Roger Poole: Trade union official whose impeccable public persona helped ambulance workers defeat the Tory government', *The Independent.* https://www.independent.co.uk/news/people/news/roger-poole-trade-union-official-whose-impeccable-public-persona-helped-ambulance-workers-defeat-the-10419981.html

Quality Assurance Agency Benchmark Statements. (2019) https://www.qaa.ac.uk/docs/ qaa/subject-benchmark-statements/subject-benchmark-statement-paramedics. pdf?sfvrsn=7735c881_4

Stevens, S. (2004) 'Reform strategies for the English NHS', *Health Affairs*, 23(3), pp. 37–44.

Valderas, J. M., Starfield, B., Sibbald, B., Salisbury, C. & Roland, M. (2009) 'Defining comorbidity: Implications for understanding health and health services', *The Annals of Family Medicine*, 7(4), pp. 357–363.

van der Gaag, A. & Donaghy, J. (2013) 'Paramedics and professionalism: Looking back and looking forwards', *Journal of Paramedic Practice.* Mark Allen Group, 5(1), pp. 8–10.

Woollard, M. (2006) 'The role of the paramedic practitioner in the UK', *Journal of Emergency Primary Health Care (JEPHC)*, 4(1).

Woollard, M. (2009) 'Professionalism: Professionalism in UK paramedic practice', *Journal of Emergency Primary Health Care (JEPHC)*, 7.

# 3  Exploring the literature

## 3.1 Introduction

Literature pertaining to paramedic practice has grown steadily over the past several years. This has led to several peer-reviewed paramedic journals being formed, such as the *Journal of Paramedic Practice* (UK), the *British Paramedic Journal*, the *Emergency Medicine Journal* (EMJ), and the *Australasian Journal of Paramedic Practice*. In contrast, literature on the socialisation of ambulance workers dates to the 1980s with several seminal works influencing the field, such as Metz (1981), Palmer (1983), Mannon (1992), Reynolds (2007), McCann et al. (2013), Devenish (2014), Wankhade and Mackway-Jones (2015), Corman (2017), and the recent substantial publication by McCann (2022).

Compared to the established health professions such as nursing, physiotherapy, radiography, and so on, paramedic practice has only recently emerged to reveal new insights into how and why paramedics function in a demanding and challenging working environment. We believe it is important to review the research on areas such as culture, curriculum, pedagogy, communities of practice, enculturation, and professionalism of student paramedics and experienced paramedics, to establish a theoretical background to this book.

This chapter explores, reviews, and interrogates the literature. The principal discourses arising out of the literature shape the interpretation of subculture, since the context of the study lies within a stringent authoritarian organisation comprised of an inner-city National Health Service (NHS) ambulance service trust, along with a large university, delivering undergraduate paramedic science degree programmes. These two opposing settings present subcultures which have strong influences on paramedic development. To help illustrate the processes and experiences which face neophyte paramedics, which comprises of the formal structured paramedic university setting, with an opposing busy, unpredictable, and often chaotic clinical working environment, provides the context for the literature review. Considering this, we needed to unearth the existing literature and drill down on the concepts and how they have been used in the workplace practice. To do this, we looked at

DOI: 10.4324/9781032721408-3

the works of Corman (2017), Mannon (1992), Palmer (1983), McCann et al. (2013), Metz (1981), Devenish (2014), and Wankhade and Mackway-Jones (2015)) to help understand the concept of enculturation into the ambulance and paramedic services. The enculturation which we are proposing is the interaction between paramedic students, along with neophyte paramedics, and experienced paramedics found in their clinical workplace setting. The works of authors such as Hammersley and Atkinson (1993), O'Reilly (2009), Madden (2010), Brewer (2000), van Maanen (2011), Becker et al. (1961), Delamont (2008), and Mead (1936) subsequently add to the literature to illuminate the wider aspects of ethnography within society to help us illustrate the relationship between the formal and informal learning environments. Not surprisingly, the literature search concentrated on identifying relationships between the university classroom setting and ambulance/paramedic setting. Opposing arguments within the literature were examined, as also seen in the work of Donaghy (2010) and Devenish (2014), to help unpack and critique the possibility of student paramedics becoming enculturated into a very different traditional working environment, to that cultivated in university.

In the next section, a short summary of the various components of the chapter offers some key points from each section.

In Section 3.2, we begin by exploring culture and subculture, which is important as these terms can be used in different ways, and in order to understand the practices of the paramedic students a framework was required to adequately describe what could be going on between their practice and the university. A key finding from this section has been that practices disseminate values in a hidden way, whether that be in the university or on placement, and this led to further research on the hidden curriculum.

In Section 3.3, organisational culture is explored, as this gives rise to a form of culture often unseen by those outside the organisation of the ambulance service. A depiction of Schein's (2004) model of organisational culture acts as a scaffold to help unpack and understand how these concepts influence and inform student culture. By drawing on Schein's three-stage approach to organisational culture, we believe it can reveal how students get drawn into a very different culture to that seen in the university. A key finding emerging from this section has been that the organisational model highlights how the culture changes depending upon perceptions.

In Section 3.4, we suggest the subculture, and its underlying hidden curriculum, contributes to and inhibits student learning in the clinical practice setting (Alsubaic, 2015). The seminal works of Jackson (1968), Hafferty and O'Donnell (2014), Becker et al. (1961), and Lave and Wenger (1991) help to provide clarity that the hidden curriculum is not the learning expected or planned in the formally structured university curriculum; it is learning which is shaped by the very basis of the workplace and working environment. This phenomenon has been observed by other studies which have found students being exposed to a very different pedagogy in the clinical setting from that which they expected, as also apparent in the work of Becker et al. (1961) and

Hafferty and O'Donnell (2014). An understanding of why students and experienced paramedics appear to work within the boundaries set by a hidden curriculum is important, as the tension between the two conflicting curricula is an unexamined consequence. We will refer to these curricula as the 'formal university curriculum' and 'hidden workplace curriculum'. A key finding here is that the underlying subculture is not necessarily unique to paramedic students, as also seen in the work of Boychuck Duchscher and Cowin (2004) on newly qualified nurses.

In Section 3.5, professional identity and professionalisation are examined. The work of Devenish (2014) helps to discuss the concept of paramedic professionalism and professional identity, as he describes how concerns were raised within the Australian ambulance service and general Australian healthcare community as paramedics transferred from an in-service training model to one which is taught in universities. Devenish found a belief existed which anticipated that graduate status would provide paramedics with greater professionalism and autonomy. The study by Coster et al. (2008) identifies the extent to which students learn together and how they 'perceive' professional identity is very different. Reynolds (2007), also studying paramedic professionalism, illustrates different discourses of inter-professionalism and how these impact on professionals and service users. Reynolds (2004) reports that multiple professional identities, cloaked within the concept of professionalism, may be experienced by student paramedics as well as experienced paramedics as they become exposed to the working environment. The work of O'Meara (2011) sheds light on this, by suggesting that this is systematic within the paramedic profession, although Burford et al. (2014), on the other hand, consider the concept of professionalism of paramedics in the (UK to be too abstract to define. A key finding from this section has been that the professional identity of student paramedics and experienced paramedics is not unique, as also seen in the work of Devenish (2014) on student paramedics in Australia.

In Section 3.6, the use of paramedic storytelling is explored, something which Tangherlini (2000) aligns with the broader aspects of paramedic identity. Forms of storytelling often run counter to the dominant media representation of the paramedic field which is so often presented in many fictional and documentary representations of the working 'reality' of paramedics. These fictional representations depict very positive and harmonious relationships between crew members, ambulance managers (officers), the public, patients, and other healthcare and emergency service professionals. The often jovial and unassuming banter between crews and trainee (student) paramedics is positively portrayed. A key finding from this section revealed that this form of storytelling is unique to groups, such as paramedics.

In Section 3.7, the interpretation of pedagogy in practice, rather than skills acquisition alone, is decisive and can inform an understanding of the practice environment. By this we mean students get to learn how and when to use their newly taught skills. They can contextualise and implement these skills at the appropriate time, although this can distract them from the knowledge which they have received at the university and sets the tone for the clinical workplace. The relationship between the pedagogy experienced in the clinical workplace setting is important, as both concepts have different meanings, yet both appear inseparable for the students once they are in the workplace (Lave & Wenger, 1991). We needed to drill down, to understand the relationship between both concepts. The extent to which this can influence student paramedic pedagogy can give rise to a particular form of student enculturation into the working environment, as mentioned earlier to that found in the work (Boychuck Duchscher & Cowin, 2004) on newly qualified nurses.

In Section 3.8, various components of the workplace environment which can cause forms of tension and anxiety for students and paramedics are identified. These issues are often entwined within the nuances and intricacies of the day-to-day work and not necessarily related to the traumatic events which could reasonably be expected to impact on paramedics' anxiety and stress levels. Considering this, it was important for us to understand the issues which result from this dichotomy. A key finding from this section has highlighted that the working practices which students were expected to conform to stifled and confused students as they became caught up in a chaotic working environment.

In Section 3.9, we begin by defining enculturation. This is important as this term lies at the very essence of this thesis and is influenced by, and on, the subculture, hidden curriculum, and resulting pedagogy. As noted by Choy and Delahaye (2011), students contextualise the formal taught elements of study within the sociocultural and functional environment of the workplace. Enculturation draws on established and accepted norms and values of a particular culture or society, where accepted members fulfil the functions and roles of the group. This is also seen in the work of Gibson and Brightwell (2006) as boundaries and accepted behaviours are established, which dictates both, acceptable and unacceptable, standards of the group or society.

In Section 3.9.1, the chapter is summarised by highlighting the various national and international literature pertaining to paramedic culture in order to encapsulate, compare, and contrast the various models of student paramedic enculturation. The similarities between the various types of ambulance cultures and that of the day-to-day working subculture which students become exposed to are depicted within the relevant literature. Associated concepts within the literature are unearthed as the ramifications for practice illustrate the relationship between these concepts and enculturation. In understanding these concepts, the work draws together developments of the paramedic profession both within and outside the UK to help contextualise the paramedic landscape within the recognised body of literature. We provide this overview of the chapter to help the reader distinguish between various elements of the study. The next section looks at culture and subculture.

## 3.2 Culture and subculture

Like other constructs which we have drawn on in this book, we believe it is important here to define culture, as this is a dominant construct of this thesis which revolves around a certain form of culture. Geertz (1973: 89) defines culture as, 'inherited conceptions expressed in symbolic forms by means of which men communicate, perpetuate and develop their knowledge about and attitudes toward life'. Subculture may be defined as arising from a sub-set of culture, a small group with their norms, symbols, interactions, and language which are specific to them. Stevenson et al. (2002: 701) define this as '[t]he distinct culture of a group existing within a larger culture'.

Agnew and Kaufman (2010) and Lewis (1933) describe how a particular subculture emerged in a group of young men to form a deviant group whose potential menace on social and racial welfare formed part of their behaviours. Burt's (1925: 39–40) early work also describes young deviants as 'defective, a typical street-Arab, dull, mongos, cretins and subnormal'. The racial over-tones depicted here by Burt are at the limit of our world view. Likewise, Bell (2010) claims that early literature depicts the notion of subculture and subculturalist as having theoretical lineage with deviance. Early depiction of subculture situates the term alongside words such as deviance, defective, and non-conformist. Blackman (2014), however, describes subculture consider-ing the modern reincarnation of the term, suggesting subcultural theory has now been adapted to reflect the various sociological paradigms. In short, the term deviance is not necessarily used in this context. Furthermore, subculture is linked to fashion, such as changes within contemporary society, making the term an indicator of social and cultural measurement across centuries of change in society.

Parson's (1942) claim, that subcultural theory is a complex and prag-matic concept in relation to sociology, however, remains true. This is because the concept has since been constructed using academic and accepted usage, suggesting subculture is about different ways in which people behave and perform (Blackman, 2014). Becker (1963) and Clinard (1974), for exam-ple, found that subcultures have discrete values and cultural practices which are shared and form different cultures to that of the mainstream. Studies on emergency medical technicians (EMTs) and paramedics have found charac-teristic values and cultural practices were shared between the groups, which were different from the mainstream culture, such as those referred to by Palmer (1983), Mannon (1992), Metz (1981), and Corman (2017). Subcul-tures recognise society and culture as being distinct from, but also resistant to, the dominant culture (Blackman, 2014). For example, Metz (1981) and Mannon (1992) found a culture existed between paramedics and emergency medical technicians which was distinctive to them. They imply that crews would 'run-hot' (meaning using the ambulance's audible and visual warn-ing lights and sirens), as if on route to an emergency call, when in fact they may not be 'running- hot'. Thornton (1995: 510), referring to the work of Bourdieu, describes subculture as 'the cultural knowledge and commodities acquired by members of a group, raising their status, and helping to differentiate themselves from members of other groups'.

Paramedic students returning to university, following just a short period of clinical placement lasting two to three weeks, were seen to adopt different attitudes and behaviours from those previously seen, as also recognised in Devenish's (2014) work. We provide an extract from the original fieldnotes taken from the pilot study as an example, as students returned to university following a short period of time (two weeks) in the workplace. I recall from my notes that I questioned two female students enquiring as to how they had enjoyed their time in clinical practice. I was shocked and disappointed by the reaction of the students as a torrent of foul language and distasteful remarks followed. The following quotation taken from my fieldnotes illustrates this. For the sake of authenticity, I have kept the language used by the students (Claire and Gill).

---

Question: 'so how was your time in clinical placement-what station did you go to?'
Answer: 'it was all a fucking waste of time; we were at sunny side ambulance station and all we dealt with was a load of old shit'.

Taken from my fieldnotes (Claire & Gill 04/03/2013).

---

To help contextualise the two very different environments, university and workplace, the additional example in the following, again taken from the pilot interview with a student, helps illustrate the relationship between this paramedic student's expectations of the workplace culture and that which she experienced.

---

I was speaking to Jennie in the classroom after she had recently returned to university following her clinical practice placement. She seemed different, despondent, and fed-up. I asked her what was wrong. She spoke about the workplace culture and how we (students) must fit into this dodgy culture. She told me of working practices that she had to do, which were not taught at university. 'It's a different world out there to what we do at university', she proclaimed.

Taken from my fieldnotes (22/04/2013).

---

Whether students are aware of it or not, a subculture can influence and shape their workplace experience (Devenish, 2014). Metz (1981) found that a form of subculture existed in his early seminal ethnography of EMTs and paramedics, although it is worth noting here that, in Metz's early work, there were more EMTs than paramedics, so he focuses his study predominantly on EMTs.

He found that they worked in a vacuum, often contrary to formal policy, by doing their own thing. This meant that experienced EMTs, paramedics, and trainees would revert to the traditional taken-for-granted ways of working. To enable student paramedics to fit into the cultural context of the workplace setting, we looked at the literature pertaining to paramedics in Canada and the work of Corman (2017) who found experienced paramedics, 'old-timers', would encourage students to follow the taken-for-granted traditional practices and procedures which were then carried out by the students. The work of Becker et al. (1961) on medical students further assisted our understanding as they also discussed the distinct form of subculture which existed amongst medical students as they worked within the formal processes of the medical faculty. For example, they found students had a perceived idea of what they were about to learn in medical school and clinical practice did not coincide with those of their teachers. The following example provides an extract from the work of Becker et al. as it describes how, in orientation week, the medical fraternity hint at the workload which follows:

You start work immediately because there will be no time to catch up. Perhaps for some of you, even if you caught up, there will not be time enough. We want to keep the tension down for you. Doctors are always anxious. There are 5,000 names of parts of the body you will have to learn.

(Becker et al., 1961: 89–90)

Later in Chapter 6, examples of these are provided to help illustrate how the work of Becker et al. (1961) sheds light on the different subcultures fostered within the medical faculty and wider medical fraternity as students described not knowing what to do at the start of clinical practice. They were unaware of the unwritten rules, such as being guided by nursing colleagues, not sitting around idle, and not getting involved in areas that one is unfamiliar with. Metz's (1981) ethnography helps to illustrate the very fabric of the EMT and paramedic environment by depicting the day-to-day work of the ambulance crew. He illuminates the collegiate relationships between crews, the dark humour displayed by crews, and the trauma of the job. In trying to understand the student paramedics' clinical practice experience, we used both Becker's and Metz's work to help illustrate this point further, as Metz (1981) found EMTs and paramedics became drawn into a very traditional orthodoxy of established cultural practices, such as not stepping out of line with the more experienced crew members by just doing what they were told to do. We revisited Lave and Wenger's (1991) work, who argue that new groups are formed within the workplace setting, as opposed to the groups formed outside the work setting, such as the university. We found communities of practice contribute to an understanding of how students become drawn into the workplace setting, as various cultural groups are formulated and structured. Mead's work offers some insight into the individual's self-concept arising from the social experiences which can influence and shape their behaviour. The literature indicates that there is a potential clash of cultures between the practice and curriculum of the university and those within the ambulance services where students train. The context in which students learn is fundamental (Blackman, 2014), as Kelly (2006) suggests the classroom setting and the practice setting have significant differences. Jackson (1968) implies that two opposing settings exist, the formal and informal, which prepare students with knowledge of hierarchical power relations. Students unknowingly become exposed to the existence of a hidden curriculum because of the workplace culture which leads students to unwittingly depict a form of behaviour very different from that taught in the classroom setting. This is further depicted by Taylor and Wendland (2014) and Kramsch (1999: 111) who describe individuals as 'having difficulty relinquishing already taken-for-granted cultural perceptions, beliefs and behaviours when attempting to adapt to a new culture'. Therefore, the work of Schein launched us to try and help figure out what was happening here, as Schein (1985) highlights the subcultures which can exist in social interactions, suggesting that the very nature of the workplace can create a different set of values to that prescribed by the organisation. Wankhade (2015) provides some additional insight of an inner-city NHS ambulance service trust by highlighting how a subtle yet powerful workplace subculture existed within the ambulance service. This was very different from the culture proclaimed by senior managers of the ambulance service and academic staff. Examples of these can be found in Chapter 5. In the process of understanding student paramedics' enculturation into the ambulance service, we referred to Agnew and Kaufman (2010), Lewis (1933), and Burt (1925) who indicate that the subculture is defined by the concepts synonymous with deviancy, such as deviant (subversive) behaviours, exclusive of small group behaviours, symbols, interactions, and language, although, as previously discussed, Blackman (2014) describes deviance in contemporary society as a form of social behaviour, indicating that its etymological roots are no longer in the realm of deviancy. Building on this, we now set out a theoretical framework for addressing enculturation as it applies to a particular group of students' socialisation into the reality of the workplace culture of becoming paramedics. Here, both the formal and hidden curriculum become intensely problematic, as they can both assist and impede paramedic pedagogy. Considering the aforementioned discussions, in the next section, we draw on Schein's (1985) model of organisational culture, to help unpack the ingrained subculture which we argue exists within the ambulance service.

## 3.3 Organisational culture

Schein's (1985) model of organisational culture helps illustrate and positions this work within a theoretical framework, as he depicts three distinct constructs, to illustrate this. These constructs consist of shared values, beliefs, and various assumptions. His model illustrates how people within the organisation behave and interact with colleagues, the public, and others, how decisions are made, and how work activities are carried out, see Figure 3.1. Flamholtz and Randle (2011: 6) suggest organisation corresponds to corporate personality, which implies that every organisation, regardless of size, has a culture that influences how people behave. We went back to Schein's (1985) model to help understand the observable aspects of culture, because his model of culture infers those individual behaviours change. Whilst recognising the complexity of culture, this study acknowledges that the construction of individual professional identities may be subject to a specific cultural context, such as the culture depicted by paramedics as superheroes, such as those found in Tangherlini's (2000) work.

We depict Schein's model to symbolise three distinct components to which the culture of an organisation or institution is portrayed and provide a unique

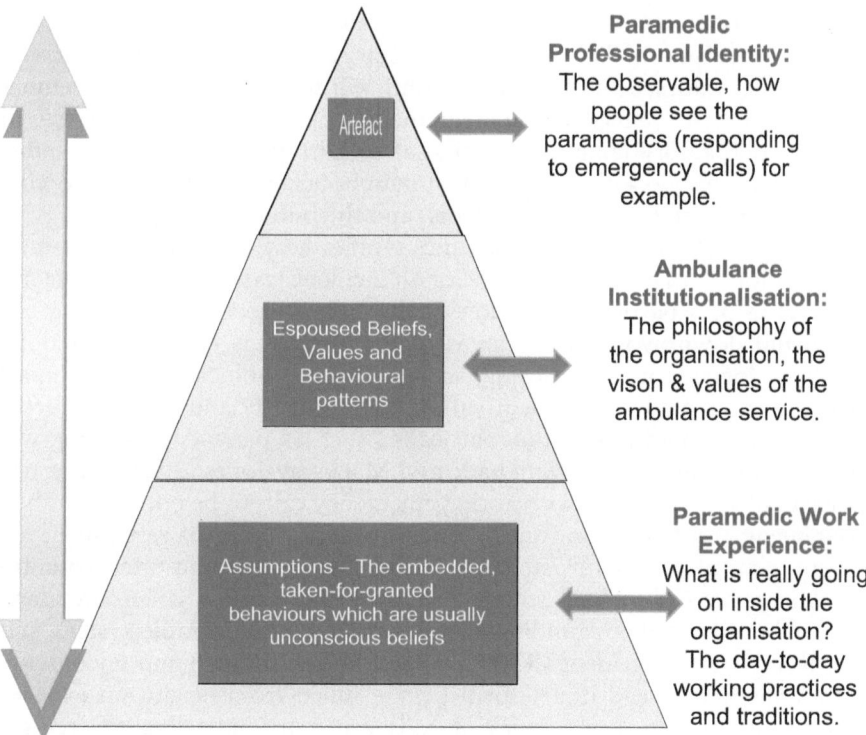

*Figure 3.1* An adaptation of Schein's (1985) model of organisational culture.

lens in which to depict the organisational culture. The first construct, arte-facts, describes how people within the organisation are seen by others outside the organisation, through their observable appearances, behaviours, com-munication, and workplace. In the context of this study, we see this as por-traying how members of the public may visualise the ambulance service, for example the blue flashing lights and sirens as the ambulance rushes through the streets as paramedic lifesavers respond to a life-threatening emergency. Similarly, McCann et al. (2013) describe organisational culture as posing the corporate values and behaviours that are expected of the organisation. Schein's second construct, espoused beliefs, consists of the values and behav-ioural patterns embedded within an organisation. We see this as how organi-sations carry out their functions, such as the way in which 999 emergency calls are responded to, how patients are treated, how the patients' clinical conditions are managed, and how patients are transported safely to hospital within the prescribed policies, procedures, and philosophy of the ambulance service. These are all fundamental tenants and values of the ambulance ser-vice and the paramedics' role within it. Schein's third construct offers an alternative view, one steeped in the day-to-day work of the people within the organisation, which we employ as those of front-line paramedics. This comprises of basic underlying assumptions, which Schein acknowledges as being what *really goes on in the organisation*. A specific type of organisa-tional culture exists here, one that forms a subculture, unseen by those out-side the organisation. This subculture comprises of forms of behaviour, such as language, values, attitudes, and customs, not seen or expected by members of the public, academics, or senior managers of the ambulance service, for example derogatory language directed at certain types of patients common throughout the workplace, sexism, homophobia, and inappropriate com-ments and innuendos to staff, students, and the public.

Palmer's (1989) study of paramedics typifies how crews would pre-judge callers prior to arriving at the scene of an incident (call), suggesting this may be because of a particular location of the call, for example attending calls to squalid downtown, shabby areas of the city, areas consisting predomi-nantly of social (council) housing, such as tenement blocks, high-rise apart-ments, and areas of social deprivation. Metz (1981) and Mannon (1992) found crews would talk about 'shit-calls', such as patients presenting with flu-like symptoms, whilst Wankhade and Mackway-Jones (2015) along with Corman (2017) found crews wanting emergency calls to be potentially about excitement and 'blood and guts'. They found a degree of resentment and stereotyping of patients existed. For example, crews would often volunteer for emergency calls which sounded exciting and serious when ambulance control broadcasted outstanding emergency calls over the radio system, such as a Road Traffic Accident (RTA) a person knocked down and unconscious with a suspected head injury, or a person fallen from height, an expected fatality and so on. These types of calls are more appealing to crews as opposed to the more mundane calls, such as an elderly person collapsing or suffering from abdominal (abdo) pains and so on. These examples provide an authentic insight into what really goes on in the organisation which helpfully depicts Schein's third construct. To further contextualise this, we went back to McCann et al. (2013), who found the organisational culture embedded within the NHS ambulance service trust where their study was conducted as authoritative and bureaucratic. This is explored in more detail later Chapter 6.

In this section of the chapter, literature pertaining to subculture has been investigated. To summarise this section and the relationships between organisational culture, culture and subculture are important in understanding the potential similarities between the cultural constructs depicted by Schein (1985), to that which applies to the workplace.

In the next section of the chapter, the hidden curriculum inherent within the workplace is explored. In doing so, we offer an understanding of how and why experienced paramedics and student paramedics resort to a form of workplace culture which is far removed from that cultivated and encouraged in university. These reveal how student paramedics display these tenancies in the workplace setting. For example, some students in the study very early on in the investigation displayed an open and transparent acceptance of the type of culture they found themselves in. They became an integral part of the workplace culture, quickly adopting the slangy informal language and behaviours of their more experienced paramedics, whilst other students were not so open and transparent. For example, these students did not openly and enthusiastically engage in the banter and rituals which formed part of the working practices of paramedic life, although Cox (2005) may argue they were an integral part of that culture, and they had just not recognised it yet.

## 3.4 Hidden curriculum

To understand how and why a subtle, yet dominant, hidden curriculum appears to form part of the paramedic students' workplace experience, we looked at Matheson (2019) work, as a variety of social interactions are experienced by paramedics and student paramedics in the practice setting. These comprise of working relationships forged between experienced paramedics, mentors, ambulance service managers, services users (patients), carers, other emergency service personnel, nursing staff, hospital staff, and members of the public, which students sometimes find challenging. Carlson et al. (2010) noted that professional socialisation may have a negative impact, as observational forms of learning can lead students to internalise poor practice. Similarly, Henderson's (2002) study of nursing provides insight into what is really going on here. Both Carlson and Henderson found nurses, in part, developed their social identity through the influences of senior role models, such as mentors and experienced staff, which they conclude was particularly evident in the way experienced staff provided care, even if this contradicted that which has been taught to the students in the classroom setting. Similar findings were reported by Greenwood (1984) and Mackintosh (2006) who described how student nurses' views and attitudes became negative after increasing exposure to clinical practice. For example:

> Nurses were more negative once they had spent time in clinical practice, citing negative examples of care or incidents where participants felt that care was missing or less than ideal by giving examples of staff who appeared to have less than caring attitudes.
>
> (Mackintosh, 2006: 957)

Campeau's (2008: 286) work on paramedics suggests 'what sets paramedics apart from nursing colleagues, is the setting in which they practice'. Campeau (2008) further argues that paramedics adapt their clinical practice into their work context; subsequently, paramedics often practise a distinctive type of care, which is that of the street, meaning paramedic work is unpredictable, not necessarily set in sterile clinical conditions or within planned procedures but rather unpredictable and chaotic. Nelson (1997: 162) finds paramedic clinical skills are often performed in a 'context rife with chaotic, dangerous, and often uncontrollable elements with which hospital-based practitioners need not contend'. Although, some accident and emergency (A&E) front-line workers, such as hospital staff, might contest this view as similar chaotic, unpredictable, and dangerous circumstances can occur within hospital departments.

Whilst Nelson (1997) illustrates the unpredictable nature of paramedic work, we were also reminded of Lipsky's (2010) ethnography of police officers in the United States of America (USA). Lipsky (2010) puts forward a similar account of the unpredictable and often challenging environments which contribute to the camaraderie he found in his study. An example could be riding out on shift with a police officer, whilst chasing a motor vehicle (car), which is eventually stopped. The apprehension and insecurity of a police officer who, after stopping the stolen vehicle, must approach and confront the driver is a result of the unpredictable nature of this type of emergency work, whilst Metz's (1981) seminal work also observes how, at that time, the point of view of EMTs and paramedics became integral to the success of new trainees. Metz (1981: 93) illustrates the fragile nature of success or failure new recruits were afforded by their experienced established colleagues, stating that the 'measure of a man or woman doing paramedic work is decided at the scene of an incident'. Back at the ambulance station, Metz recalls how the result of the trainee's performance would be discussed by the traditional old-timers. This would often contribute to the working practices experienced by the trainees in the workplace culture, which is still evident to some degree and is different from that taught in the university classroom setting. Jackson (1968) implies student learning is influenced by aspects of the hidden curriculum. We were reminded of Bourdieu's (1990) work, and the similarities around subculture with forms of deviance, a phenomenon already discussed, although (Blackman, 2014) further suggests this notion is outdated, prejudiced, and fundamentally wrong today. Furthermore, Blackman (2014) offers the concept of subculture as less associated with such negative aspects of society. If this is true, then the subculture which we are proposing exists, characterised by paramedics avoiding meal breaks, avoiding finishing shifts late, avoiding certain emergency calls, and causing unnecessary damage to ambulances, along with the nuances and intricacies of the working environment, resulting from a sustained and familiar workplace subculture. It could be argued that specific types of deviant behaviours are going on here which have become part of the paramedic subculture, such as institutional deviance.

The diverse nature of paramedic work, noted by Palmer (1989) and Corman (2017), accompanied with the desire for students to fit-in to the established culture identified by Becker et al. (1961), manifests from past practices and traditions, resulting in a particular type of pedagogy. This pedagogy is complex and integral to the hidden curriculum which students experience and which is shaped by the prevailing subculture. As Devenish (2014) infers, this form of pedagogy influences student paramedics' enculturation. Lave and Wenger (1991) suggest workplace practice is contextual to the practice environment in which it is situated, whilst Strauss and Quinn (1997) argue that cultural influences contribute to the learning environment which are based on recurring common experiences, mediated by learned practices in the practice placement setting.

Students become enculturated into a complex web of workplace practices which they struggle to understand. The unfamiliar educational process which confronts them in the clinical workplace setting is challenging. Devenish's (2014: 13) findings, in part, act as a foundation to our work, as he found students 'did not appear to understand the ambulance culture, similarly many paramedics were not familiar with university culture'. Significant numbers of experienced paramedics in the UK and Australian workforce may not necessarily possess a university education because the ambulance services were previously formed from a very traditional manual working environment, as identified by McCann et al. (2013). This leads to a hidden curriculum formed from established and taken-for-granted ways of working and traditions. Hafferty (1998) and O'Donnell (2014) consider these ways of working as being responsible for the learning which occurs outside the formal curriculum, which Hafferty (2014: 7) suggests is '[t]he place one learns, often tacitly, how things work around here'. What is taken from this is that the day-to-day pedagogy which students are exposed to is far removed from that envisaged by the academic community, professional and regulatory bodies, and ambulance service managers. Similar findings are seen in McCann et al. (2013), Wankhade and Mackway-Jones (2015), and Reynolds (2004) work, where the structure and culture of the ambulance service became grounded in a very ridged, authoritarian organisation. This suggests that a paradox exists between front-line ambulance crews and managers, resulting in little understanding and appreciation of each other's roles and responsibilities.

Student paramedics are exposed to a very formal structured taught curriculum, whilst attending university, as also seen in Woollard's (2009) work. Kelly (2006) and Stenhouse (1975), discussing the same issue in schools, identify this curriculum as one that is set out by formally agreed syllabi, prospectuses, course outlines, and assessment strategies. The curriculum found outside the formal processes, however, is also what pupils really experience. What Kelly (2006) and Stenhouse (1975) infer here is that student experiences outside the formal institution, such as the school playground or workplace, can be very different from the curriculum taught within the institution. Therefore, the hidden curriculum which students are exposed to forms part of the socialisation process, which in turn results in the enculturation into the ambulance service. To understand how this hidden curriculum is experienced in the workplace and drawn from a subculture, the work of Metz (1981), Mannon (1992), Devenish (2014), and Corman (2017) helps, as paramedics and EMTs are unwittingly drawn into a subculture and subsequently a hidden curriculum. The initial findings from the pilot study are considered to help contextualise these claims. An example from the pilot study is provided here to help illustrate this point:

> James, the student paramedic, and I were on a nightshift together. Jim, the experienced paramedic was running late for work so James and I were in the crew room waiting for Jim to arrive. I was interested in how James was reluctant to talk about university in front of other paramedics in the crew room, instead wanting to engage with their conversation which was around nuisance callers, and callers that were a waste of time. It felt as though I was embarrassing James by talking about university. I thought this was reflective of a subculture which harnessed a form of a hidden curriculum which James just had to be part off.
>
> Taken from my fieldnotes (12/06/2013).

Corman (2017: 26) also recalls a time when he entered the building (ambulance station), and he says hello to Julie, who is reclining in the armchair polishing her boots. She says, 'It's going to be a good day today; someone is going to die'. She explains that whenever she polishes her boots someone dies. Corman explains that perhaps she wanted him to see a good call. Paramedics orientate to different social characteristics depending on the patient they are attending and would often pre-judge the work.

> Hanna (paramedic) guessed a patient was a heavy drinker, as she explains how 'She's uh, she's um, she's poor hygiene, she stays at the drop-in centre, and just from, well not that everybody who has those things is a heavy drinker but just from experience with this kind of clientele that I can guess',
>
> (Corman, 2017: 65)

Mannon (1992: 132) reminds us how he found EMTs and paramedics in the USA often displayed a sense of frustration and tension when they attended certain calls, he explains, 'all the bullshit you see in the districts, in part, the taxi service function', referring to how crews would perceive certain calls which they have attended, as a free taxi service. A view often shared by ambulance crews in the UK (see Chapter 5). Metz (1981) found EMTs and paramedics had widespread agreement amongst themselves about how patients should be classified and how the various classifications should be treated. Metz (1981: 113) explains, 'in other words, the EMTs and paramedics stereotype the patients and pass these attitudes along to trainees, with the result that the stereotypes become institutionalised'. This is an important claim, which further reinforces the argument that the relationship between the concepts of subculture and hidden curriculum allows them to gain specific types of informal learning, as also noted by Jackson (1968). This learning impacts on their enculturation into the workplace setting. The similarity of the students' observed behaviours, noted by Palmer (1989) and Metz (1981), may explain how and why student paramedics get drawn into the role of an actor, depicting a calm, confident, controlled individual at the scene of an incident, whilst other members of public around them are in crisis and despair. This is a very different depiction from that portrayed by students and paramedics once they are alone in the rig (ambulance). Palmer (1989) further describes how paramedics strut their stuff, by acting out the role of their more experienced colleagues. To try and answer this, we went back to Schein's (1985) model of organisational culture to help signal the very different cultures which exist. This can be one which depicts a somewhat improper, tasteless display, brought about in the confines of the ambulance or the ambulance station or other private areas, to that displayed and recognised by the public. These types of behaviours, presented by paramedics, are further seen in the works of other researchers, such as Lipsky (2010), Metz (1981), Corman (2016), Mannon (1992), Palmer (1989), Tangherlini (2000), and McCann et al. (2013). To help illustrate this, the two examples here extracted from our early exploratory fieldnotes highlight how these behaviours manifest themselves through the paramedic subculture.

Whilst I was riding out with Ben, the student paramedic, we were talking about his work at university, where I was one of his tutors. Ben is a keen, hardworking and conscientious student at university, always willing to help his peers and staff alike. Yet I was surprised by Ben's behaviour and attitude in the practice setting. I watched Ben, mimic his mentor, (experienced paramedic), not wanting to appear keen, or enthusiastic but settled to adopt a no-do culture. Such as mimicking and moaning about certain calls (jobs) derogatory comments regarding break times and finishing times and a general dismissive attitude toward ambulance control. I spoke to Ben a couple of times about his university studies whilst we were driving back to station. Ben's response was 'yeah they're okay I suppose, I do what I need to do, you know'. He then smiled at his mentor followed by a quiet giggle of laughter.

Taken from my fieldnotes (14/01/2013).

This particular shift, I was riding out with Julie, the student paramedic and Joe, the experienced paramedic. We arrived on scene at the next call, and whilst we are waiting to gain access into the premises via an intercom system on the communal door of a care home, I noticed Julie, constantly texting via her mobile phone, expressing little if any concept of her surroundings or the voice which answered the intercom. I nudged Julie to draw her attention to the fact that someone was answering the intercom system and was trying to let us in. Her colleague (Joe) was bringing the carry chair from the ambulance and as such wasn't with us at that point. This was such a different behaviour to that witnessed by the student back in university.

Taken from my fieldnotes (05/05/2013).

The subculture which we are arguing exists within the ambulance work-place is pragmatic, insular, and untenable for the future development of the modern paramedic practitioner. Hafferty and O'Donnell (2014: 18) suggest that 'distinct differences exist from the curriculum presented by the educational institutions to the curriculum which actually takes place on the shop floor'. Tindall, also referring to curricula, offers an alternative reflective interpretation of the hidden curriculum, one rooted in the distinction between one's intention and one's actions, which he illustrates as '[a] lesson in how to behave which is neither planned nor discussed' (Tindall, 1975: 2–28). For Becker et al. (1961), the lineage is more direct, claiming:

The influence of social stratification, social class, social status, and the role of place on student education and learning, contributes to a subsequent latent culture and the existence of a student culture in medical school.

(Becker et al., 1961: 304–313)

Additional two examples are provided in the following from Becker's work which we have summarised to help reinforce this point and depict the behaviour and tensions which he witnessed whilst researching medical students' workplace practice curricula and their already taken-for-granted groups or communities. Becker found that the students would finally co-operate together to avoid making a bad impression on the faculty. Becker et al. (1961: 307) also illustrate how 'they (medical students) will do another man's work for him, when circumstances make it impossible for him to do it himself; in this way they protect him from the adverse judgment the faculty would otherwise make'. Becker recalls how students received their information regarding their clinical placements, and he found they became apprehensive, anxious, and defensive of their potential separation from the group which had been shaped during their time together in the medical school. The main point from this highlights how students had become enculturated into the very fabric of the academic medical fraternity, and how they became communities of their own practice (Lave & Wenger, 1991) forming and shaping a coherent group, who then found it challenging and unsettling to leave the group, as students go from formal academic studies into a challenging, unpredictable, and often hostile working environment, which Lave and Wenger suggest:

> On the one hand, newcomers need to engage in existing practices in order to understand, participate and to become full members of the community. On the other hand, they have a stake in the development of their communities as they begin to establish their identity.
>
> (Lave & Wenger, 1991: 36)

Lipsky (2010) highlights how public sector workers in the USA, such as public housing officers, police officers, prison officers, and hospital staff, often felt restricted by formal reports, policies, and rules. Workers formed collegiate groups and would circumnavigate and bypass formal rules which they felt restricted and somewhat prohibited their working day. He notes how the traditional working customs and practices of the day-to-day work of police officers were conducted, finding this to be in sharp contrast to that laid down by formal rules and expectations from the police service managers.

> Street-level bureaucrats work in isolation, but they seek and receive support from other workers. Street-level bureaucrats are no less peer-related than other works and find gratification in the squad room, teachers' lounge, and other places where they congregate.
>
> (Lipsky, 2010: 76)

The aforementioned extract taken from Lipsky (2010) gives an indication of the subculture, along with the hidden curriculum which gives rise to it. Notwithstanding this, we found educationalists, such as Cottingham et al. (2008), refer to various terms to describe the hidden curriculum, such as informal curriculum, tacit curriculum, unintentional curriculum, and unwritten curriculum. It has also been suggested that these curricula result in working practices and traditions far removed from that taught in the formal curriculum often found in the classroom setting (Hafferty, 1998; Cowell, 1972; O'Donnell, 2014). Doja et al. (2016) found several themes which medical students identified within the hidden curriculum, and a culture of tolerance towards unprofessional behaviours and the importance of role modelling in professional identity were common. Wilkinson et al. (2016) consider that this represents a powerful and influential component to the students' educational development. Graduate paramedic students enter an established tradition of working customs and practices which often consist of behaviours not expected nor planned for by the student. We illustrate some of these practices to contextualise the impact these practices can have on the ambulance service and student pedagogy. These practices include behaviours such as avoiding emergency calls where possible, excessive downtime (unavailability for calls) whilst at hospitals, and avoiding late finishes and meal breaks. Occasionally this includes more sinister behaviours, such as damaging ambulance vehicles (see Chapter 5). Students find these practices and traditions difficult to understand, in part, as these components of practices are not shared, nor spoken of, whilst students are in the university.

Mead (1936) found people can adapt and adjust to the social structure and behaviours. These can consist of copying or falling in line with other people's behaviours, such as the more experienced paramedics (old-timers), suggesting student paramedics have little control over the social structure of the workplace as this has previously been mapped out by the existing behaviours, customs, and norms of the traditional working practices. Becker et al. (1961), describing medical students' induction into medical school, found students expected a scripted formal form of pedagogy, although this was not what students found in their practice sessions. Hafferty and O'Donnel (2014) describe the type of behaviour found in the healthcare setting as being common practice throughout the workforce.

Jackson (1968), Dreeben (1968), and Vallance (1986) provide a deeper understanding of the emergence of the hidden curriculum. They suggest it is implicit in many guises that the curriculum outside these parameters becomes the unwritten curriculum or hidden curriculum. They further suggest that any formal curriculum is often accompanied by an opposing curriculum which sits outside of formal control. In this case, the hidden curriculum provides a form of pedagogy which is neither planned, nor spoken of, in the students' formal university studies. This, it would seem, knowingly or unknowingly, exposes students to a form of pedagogy which is scripted within the traditional ways, customs, and norms of the working environment, as set out by the experienced traditional workforce.

The following examples depict the formal university curricula, taught to paramedic students, in one university, along with an example of the statutory regulatory requirements expected of paramedics. In addition, an early sample of data taken from our exploratory fieldnotes offers a contextualisation of the fragmented environment in which paramedics operate.

Extract taken from the University of Hertfordshire Paramedic Curriculum (2020):

> This module has been designed to provide you (students) with insight into the current role of the paramedic and associated disciplines, along with the future of the Paramedic profession. It relates to other modules on your course as it threads through all areas of the paramedic role and furthermore has been designed to support you to think beyond tradition and consider the pathway your own career may take. The module hopes to inspire Paramedic students to continue into postgraduate study and play an active role in the development of the Paramedic profession.
>
> (University Module Content – The Professional Role of the Paramedic, 2020)

Extract taken from the HCPC's Standards of Proficiency.

1.4 be able to work safely in challenging and unpredictable environments, including being able to take appropriate action to assess and manage risk
2.3 understand the need to respect and uphold the rights, dignity, values, and autonomy of service users including their role in the diagnostic and therapeutic process and in maintaining health and wellbeing
3.1 understand the need to maintain high standards of personal and professional conduct
5.2 understand the need to demonstrate sensitivity to the factors which shape lifestyle that may affect the individual's health and the interaction between the service user and paramedic
6.0 Be able to practice in a non-discriminatory manner

(Standards of Proficiency for Paramedics, 2023)

---

We arrived at hospital and handed over our patient, whilst Julian (Paramedic) completed the paperwork in the front cab of the ambulance. I noticed he leant back in his seat and put his feet up on the dashboard deliberately kicking the air vent until it was shattered in pieces, before kicking it again and breaking the last remaining piece of plastic. He seemed unconcerned by the amount of damage he was causing and just continued to get comfortable and push his feet into the air vent causing even more damage.

Taken from my fieldnotes (13/04/2013).

> (Q) 'Is there anything you want to tell me that would assist me in my research' (Last Question).
>
> (A) 'Yeah, well its different out there (clinical practice), I think a lot of us (students) when we get in practice are okay but sometimes it just takes time to know where you need to be, you know to fit in, as opposed to you are just in it like that. I think they (experienced paramedics) are generally okay but do things different from what we have been taught, err you know short cuts and stuff like that'.
>
> Extract from early exploratory student interview with Charles (03/10/2013).

We argue that these perspectives of recurrent behaviours, like those highlighted in the two previous examples, become endemic throughout the workplace and act as the students' customary approach to the workplace setting, as also experienced by Becker et al.'s (1961) ethnography of medical students, Metz's (1981) ethnography of EMTs and paramedics, and Mannon's (1992) work of EMTs and paramedics, along with Devenish's (2014) work on student paramedics in Australia. In addition, Corman's (2017) ethnography of Canadian paramedics provides a degree of confidence that these practices and behaviours are also to be found in his seminal works. Hundert (1996) also raises concerns that the hidden curricula may be found in many levels of organisations or institutions, such as educational establishments, commerce, and industry, arguing that this is a consequence of rigid structures and formal rules and policies which subsequently influence behaviours and working practices. The policies and rules which Hundert (1996) refers to are not conducive of the day-to-day work found in the ambulance service or that which Lipsky (2010) highlights in his study of housing officers and police officers.

The work of Bray (2017), examining the hidden curriculum in schooling, believes the hidden curriculum may now have reached a point at which it is no longer hidden. The two juxtapositions, formal and informal (hidden curriculum), become evident, as students are drawn into a silo of fitting into the traditional orthodoxy of working practices and behaviours. The powerful and influential nature of the hidden curriculum means that some students become detached from their future professional aspirations and developments. For example, very early in the investigations we found that students were not necessarily concerned about becoming an advanced paramedic, specialist paramedic, primary care practitioner, flight paramedic, or critical care paramedic (COP, 2019). Instead, some students continued to work in the confines of the unintentional hidden curriculum as students became focused on fitting-in with their experienced colleagues. This is how students start to get drawn into a community of practice which Lave and Wenger's (1991) work clearly depicts. The work of O'Donnell (2014) examines the impact of student behaviour, believing the knowledge and experience expected of students exposed to the practice setting are often limited and aligned to the subculture, suggesting that this is implicit within the clinical setting of medical education. Anyon (1981), Giroux (2001), and Vallance (1986) believe this remains consistent throughout education, indicating the hidden curriculum orchestrates many sociocultural aspects of society. Paramedic students are restricted, restrained, and unable to use their newly taught theories, knowledge, and skills in the practice setting. This is an unintended and negative consequence of the hidden curriculum which Ball (2005) goes some way to help illustrate:

> Holistic ways of working which take a far wider approach to service provision are the long-term goal therefore and, as such, must impact upon the future training of the paramedic. Paramedic training must move its focus away from the acquisition of clinical skills (no matter how wide ranging), towards fostering the ability to think and practice autonomously. In the short term, paramedics must be taught to appropriately diagnose and manage a wider range of patients, practically those who present with hidden conditions, minor illnesses, and minor trauma. In the longer term, and more importantly however, they must learn to work together to take ownership of the basic philosophies of their practice, which are solidly grounded in the methodologically valid and reliable research, and therefore truly evidence based.
>
> (Ball, 2005: 899)

Ball (2005) advocates for an advanced curriculum to support the concept of paramedic development, which the hidden curriculum and the corresponding subculture impede and hamper. The 2008 report on the Pre-Registration Education and Funding for Paramedics (DH, 2008) helped to provide a sense to move to higher education, suggesting this is crucial if the paramedic profession is to meet the future demands and requirements of the employer and increasing public expectations. An extract of this is illustrated here:

> Health Education England's (HEE) major piece of work stemming from the 2014 publication of the Paramedic Evidence Based Education Project, which recommended the introduction of a single point of education entry at degree level for paramedic training. The Paramedic Education and Training Steering Group was established to review the potential benefits of up skilling and training paramedics to enable them to deliver more treatment in the community, as well as better delivery of on-site triage and treatment in emergencies, where clinically appropriate.
>
> (DH, 2008)

However, it is unclear and difficult to quantify from the evidence just how successful and influential the introduction of an all-graduate profession has been in shaping and changing current behaviours, values, and practices of the paramedic profession, although we believe this research contributes to the literature on paramedic enculturation.

In this section, the literature on culture and education provides an understanding of the relationship between these two paradigms and student paramedics as they enter the workplace. The emphasis has been on the balance between the educational needs of student paramedics, with that of the culture, which they experience in the workplace, whereby students mirror the behaviour of the experienced traditional workforce. This appears endemic throughout the student community, as a failure to do so results in rejection from the practice community, likened by Lave and Wenger (1991) to communities of practice. To sum up the pertinent points in this section, along with their implication for practice, many of the points raised have negative connotations for practice.

To summarise this section of the chapter, we propose that an established traditional way of working, rather than the one which has been shaped and developed over time, is borne out by the work of Metz (1981), Mannon (1992), Devenish (2014), Palmer (1989), and Corman (2017). The implications for practice would suggest the profession remains restricted, stagnant, and static in its professional development, whilst a hidden curriculum is drawn out of the subculture, as also highlighted by Anyon (1981), Giroux (2001), Vallance (1986), O'Donnell (2014), and Hafferty (2014). This produces student paramedics who replicate the traditional ways and behaviours of previous years producing a pedagogy which is steeped in the traditional, taken-for-granted, ways of working, as the two opposing curriculums are formed. The implications for practice stem from inconsistencies which students may experience in both their clinical practice experience and educational experience. The formal university curriculum does not accurately reflect the hidden curriculum which students become exposed to in the practice setting.

In the next section of this chapter, literature pertaining to professional identity and professionalism within the ambulance service is discussed. This is important and adds to this research, as the notion of professionalism can have a significant influence over the traditional behaviours and customs embedded within the traditional workplace environment.

## 3.5  Paramedic professionalism and professional identity

In this section, professionalism and paramedic professional identity is, to an extent, an abstract concept in the context of paramedics, as often mooted and debated within the literature. The work of Burford (2012), Donaghy (2010), McCann et al. (2013), Devenish (2014), Williams and Webb (2015),

Lovegrove and Davis (2013), and van der Gaag and Donaghy (2013) launches the abstract notion of professional identity in paramedic practice. Becker et al.'s (1961) study of medical students provides a helpful example of why this appears to be the case, as they found freshman students entering the medical profession became somewhat disillusioned with the medical practices which were being taught to them, viewing them as anything but professional. Williams and Webb (2015), along with Kell and Owen (2008), propose that a somewhat vague, confused understanding of the terms professional and professionalism exists. They suggest contemporary society has seen the term 'professional', as a vocational structure emerging, which can be deeply contested and which varies across geographical, cultural, and historical context. In short, as Kell and Owen (2008) have pointed out, the term professionalism has become a commonly accepted term which can be influenced by historical content, social practices, demographics, and context. At the same time, Evetts (2003: 407) suggests 'the examination of the role of HEIs in shaping paramedics professional identity reflects the increasingly ambiguous nature of professionalism in Allied Health Professions (AHPs) practice'. The meaning of professionalism is not fixed as various connotations of professionalism are required to understand the role of universities in facilitating change. Burford (2012) study of professionalism of paramedics and social workers provides a context in which to illustrate the notion of professionalisation within the UK paramedic profession, suggesting the locus of professionalism as a construct is an abstract concept to which individuals subscribe. Burford (2012) implies that the notion of professionalism remains attached to the individual despite the environment or social status. A degree of confusion and ambiguity exists amongst both students and experienced paramedics as they grapple to contextualise the concept of professionalism. Paramedic professionalisation remains embryonic and continually changing, due, in part, to the introduction of university degree programmes, as seen in the work of Donaghy (2010), statutory regulation, and membership of a professional body. The following examples help illustrate this point:

---

(Q) 'How professional did you feel the clinical practice experience was'
(A) 'Oh fuck, oops sorry John (researcher), not at all. Christ, crews didn't give a toss about that, they just wanted to do as little as possible for the most money available (overtime) and get off work and get home. I don't think it is very professional at all if you ask me'.

Extract taken from initial exploratory student interviews (pilot study with Tom 08/01/2013).

---

I was riding out with Tony, an experienced paramedic and mentor, when I asked him what he thought of the British Paramedic Association (BPA), now the College of Paramedics (professional body) and the Health Professions Council (HPC), now the HCPC (the regulatory body). Tony couldn't distinguish between the two of them and was unaware of each other's roles, responsibilities and functions, as he thought they were both: 'a bit of a waste of time I think'. Tony had little if any insight into the roles and functions of these two organisations, although as a paramedic he has a mandatory annual subscription for registration with the HCPC.

Taken from my fieldnotes (10/01/2013).

Williams and Webb (2015), Lovegrove and Davis (2013), McCann et al. (2013), Burford (2012), and van der Gaag and Donaghy (2013) consider the evidence around professionalism in the paramedic discipline, which remains unclear. A key component of the findings relies on data regarding paramedics fitness to practice (FTP) referrals (complaints against paramedics), submitted to the regulatory body, the HCPC, which increase exponentially year on year. This would indicate that paramedics are, what McCann et al. (2013) call, 'blue collar professionals', a term to describe semi-professional attitudes and behaviours, whilst Paramedics' fitness to practice cases forwarded to the HCPC remains high.

The Paramedic Evidence Based Education Project (PEEP) (Lovegrove & Davis, 2013) report suggests that paramedic development is a key component of the professionalisation agenda. We were mindful that the PEEP report lays the professionalisation agenda firmly at university education. The report suggests that, once students graduate and become paramedics, they are autonomous practitioners and able to deliver effective care. Lovegrove and Davis (2013: 7) suggest that 'for this situation to be realised, a more robust education and training system needs to be in place'. Newton's work helped us understand this a little more. Newton (2012: 12) believes 'what is needed for the modern ambulance service is a new guiding principle based on a more clinical decision focused approach'. Drawing on a professional paramedic workforce, consisting of additional clinical capabilities, Newton goes on to add, 'It is recognised that education of this workforce is essential for lasting change and is the core enabler for changing clinical behaviour' (Newton, 2012: 8). This implies that paramedic professional identity is dependent on individual perceptions and agency, such as public perception or organisational image, which Burford et al. (2014), McCann et al. (2013), and Lovegrove and Davis (2013) also infer.

Furthermore, Burford et al. (2014) found variations of expectations existed between paramedic students, their university lecturers, and their workplace colleagues, such as experienced staff. Becker et al. (1961) also illustrate how freshman students had different expectations from that of the faculty. These differences are recursive and connote attitudes towards professionalism which Burford et al. (2014) imply remain blurred. Furthermore, Lovegrove and Davis (2013) found paramedics, and student paramedics, orientate towards a strong workplace identity. These workplace identities are formed within the complexity of social, demographic, locational, or situational factors, as Corman (2016) found these identities were changed or modified depending on the social setting. Looking at the professional values of emergency services, Nurok and Henckes (2009: 9) found social categories, such as 'age, sex, race and socio-economic status', influenced and potentially mediated the care provided to patients. Pratt et al. (2006) offer an alternative concept, by reiterating the importance of knowing what people do, which will help galvanise a richer appreciation of who they are in the identity construction of professionals. For example, providing feedback and role models which Pratt et al. (2006) claim serves to improve and understand professional identity which is not the same as that fostered and nurtured in university. Metz (1981) found identity of EMTs and paramedics was an essential component of their working day. Not surprisingly, students and paramedics construct their identity through the various forms of day-to-day work, such as discursive conversations, the insignia worn on their uniforms, symbols, and personalised utility belts, which are large belts used by crews to add several utility pouches and tools such as torches, scissors, and forceps. This, in part, constructs the group's identity and helps consolidate their unique community of practice.

The difficulty is that paramedics continue to enact subtle forms of institutional work, meaning they continue to work as they have been doing for many years. An example of this can be seen as crews responding to 999 emergency calls often rotate, as opposed to decisions about who should attend being based on the clinical significance of the incident or event. For instance, when two or three ambulances are in the ambulance station and a 999 emergency call is received from ambulance control, it is usually the first ambulance in station from the previous call who responds to the next call. This is regardless of the skill set of the crew, i.e., EMTs or paramedics. The consequence of this traditional way of working may lead to a less experienced and clinically qualified ambulance crew attending a serious clinical situation, whilst the more experienced and clinically competent paramedic remains in station. We provide this example to help depict one of the traditions embedded within an often stagnant, inactive, and arguably passive workforce, which Givati et al. (2018: 353) imply, in part, is 'responsible for the complex nature of the relationship between the university and professional practice'.

This traditional workplace culture remains inherently notable throughout practice and serves to maintain a form of institutionalisation as identified by McCann et al. (2013) and further supported by Corman (2017). Paramedics and student paramedics are unclear, unsure, and unknowing of their professional identity, which Ginsberg et al. (2000) further support, suggesting professionalism remains an emerging contextualised interaction of individuals. An example from Burford et al. (2014: 3) helps illustrate this, as they observed that 'values may occasionally come into conflict, and the ultimate choice the student makes will depend on the specifics of the situation'. Paramedic workplace culture is extensively incumbent on individual agency, whereby individuals may display a form of professional behaviour in one situation, yet not in another. Aultman et al. (2009) and Kell and Owen (2008) depict this kind of professional behaviour as being inherently linked to social agency, and a mishmash of understanding becomes prevalent as students and experienced paramedics seek assurance of their professional identity. We reminded ourselves of Burford et al.'s (2014) work, who consider that this underlying complexity is what challenges professionalism as a practical concept. Boundaries between professionalism and non-professionalism remain blurred and unclear.

We conclude this section of the chapter by suggesting professionalism within paramedic practice remains an abstract concept. As Burford et al. (2014: 7) claim, '[p]rofessionalism remains conceptually unclear'. To define the notion of professionalism as an embedded construct within paramedic practice is limited, as recognised in the literature. It is embryonic in its development, evolution, and augmentation. Furthermore, as suggested by Kell and Owen (2008), it is influenced by many factors, such as the social situation, demographics, location, and circumstances.

In the next section of this chapter, the notion of storytelling as a means of communication between student paramedics and experienced paramedics, along with other emergency services, is explored. The literature on paramedic storytelling is focused on the day-to-day communication which is widespread across the profession. The language used is often derogatory and seemingly callous, yet it is embedded within paramedic practice. Traces of such can be seen in several studies (Metz, 1981; Corman, 2016; McCann et al., 2013; Mannon, 1992; Palmer, 1989; Tangherlini, 2000; Scott, 2007), which we discuss within this section.

## 3.6 Paramedic storytelling

Tangherlini's (2000) work, *Heroes and Lies: Storytelling Tactics among Paramedics*, depicts an entrenched and cynical self-deprecatory storytelling tradition which is prevalent within the practice setting of paramedics. This storytelling often runs counter to media representations of paramedics so often presented in many fictional and documentary broadcasts, for example television fictional broadcasts, such as (*Casualty*, 1986), (*Holby City*, 1999), (*Chicago Fire*, 2012), along with representations such as (*Rescue 911*, 1989) featuring re-enactments along with actual footage of emergencies which are dramatised and represented as being exciting dramatic events, whereby paramedics heroically arrive on scene in their gleaming shining rig (ambulance) along with their smartly pressed paramedic uniforms. Other examples include

*Inside the Ambulance* (2020) illustrating the work of paramedics in an often busy, caring, and unpredictable environment. Another example of this is the television broadcast *Junior Paramedics* (2014), a depiction of a very content, happy, and enthusiastic group of student paramedics going about their day-to-day work in emergency ambulances, dealing with various incidents in a supportive and friendly working environment. These depictions are in addition to media coverage of real-life situations, such as major incidents, large-scale terrorist incidents, and assaults on high-profile individuals. Paramedics, along with other emergency service personnel, are often featured and represented by the media as heroic lifesaving professionals, which in many cases they are. However, our findings would suggest another version of the 'truth' exists, despite media coverage. Both Tangherlini (2000) and Reynolds (2007) depict paramedics as a more belligerent group of individuals who often use unscrupulous and at times offensive storytelling as part of their day-to-day activities whilst working together in the rig (ambulance). The following example by Tangherlini gives an indication of the type of storytelling used by paramedics.

> deeply cynical and self-deprecatory storytelling tradition, one that countermands the media representations of their field so neatly presented in globally popular television programmes'. Rather than depicting the paramedic as silent heroes just doing our job, highlighted in media representations.
>
> (Tangherlini, 2000: 43)

Tangherlini (2000: 449) found that paramedics tended to present themselves through their stories as anti-heroes. 'They were always ready with a sardonic quip in even the most horrific situations' believing this, 'is a result of the tactical resistance to the various groups with whom they encounter on a daily basis'. This is also seen in the work of Young (1995: 151) on policing, who reveals the 'complexity of one small area of police culture which is often hidden from the outsider; for the stories about "bad" deaths and the savage black humour these generate'.

To understand this, we first went back to Lave and Wenger (1991), who highlight the context in which groups of individuals are potentially drawn together within the workplace and are identified to offer some interpretation of the paramedics' storytelling. We found that the relationship between Lave and Wenger's (1991) model of communities of practice, to some extent, became a catalyst for the various stories which paramedics used in their day-to-day work. Tangherlini's (2000) study of paramedics in the USA implies that there was a cultural ideology which influenced the behaviours and interactions of paramedics. An example of this is provided here:

> The medic's tactical resistance to the various groups of patients with whom they come into contact on a daily basis, are qualitatively different from their relationships with medical personnel, managers and

other emergency providers. Many patients and members of the public have expectations derived from 'reality television' and are often angered when medics do not behave like their television counterparts.

(Tangherlini, 2000: 59)

Tangherlini (1998: 86) further states that '[i]n the course of this storytelling, paramedics often resort to strong language, vying against each other to tell the best story'. Furthermore, Corman (2016) finds this style of storytelling pervasive and suggests that this occurred mostly in the ambulance station, or in the rig (ambulance), which may suggest this type of storytelling is used as a way of coping with the stress and angst which paramedics experience in their day-to-day work. Corman (2016) explains this storytelling by trying to understand what paramedics actually do and why, suggesting this is a characteristic of the paramedics' working environment which is unseen and unknown by their patients and the wider public. The use of slang, abbreviations, antidotes, colloquialisms, and discursive terms is identified. Terms such as truck instead of ambulance, brown-bread referring to dead, punter instead of patient, sickie meaning unwell patient (often a child), and purple-plus referring to a deceased patient who would be beyond resuscitation are commonly used in the clinical practice setting. This provides a realistic and authentic insight into the traditional workplace culture experienced by students. As referred to previously, McCann et al.'s (2013) study of paramedics in an inner-city NHS ambulance service illustrates how the tension between middle-ranking managers (officers) of the ambulance service and front-line paramedics and student paramedics became deeply precarious, which also leads to additional forms of dialogue about the fragile relationship between crew staff and managers. The following example is taken from our pilot study.

---

Whilst a paramedic crew were completing their essential patient report form at the hospital. I recall from my early pilot study fieldnotes, how the crew were then subsequently instructed by an ambulance officer to contact ambulance control to attend another call, leaving little, if any time, for the documentation to be completed sufficiently. The crew rebelled using offensive language and finding a reason not to attend the call.

Taken from my fieldnotes (01/04/2013).

---

In the light of the discussions and the example provided here, we drew on Boychuck Duchscher and Cowin's (2004) study of nurses in North America to help provide some insight into the conflict which they found between nurses and managers. They found that nurses became disadvantaged and discriminated against when in clinical practice, because senior staff bullied and intimidated newly qualified and trainee nurses. Boychuck Duchscher and Cowin's (2004) findings of student nurses provide similarities with that of student paramedics as illustrated in our study. Mulder et al.'s (2019) study explores how nurses become drawn into a hidden curriculum, whilst Kramer (1974) finds nurses are 'shocked' into the realities of the workplace. Referring to McCann et al.'s (2013) work, it reiterates the distinctive and unhelpful relationship they found existed between senior members of the ambulance service and those of the front-line paramedic workforce. At the same time, the Care Quality Commission (2015), the regulator of health and adult social services in England, found a lack of support from management within the NHS ambulance service trust where our study was conducted.

To understand why the paramedic workplace proved so challenging, we reviewed the literature on cultural identity and the work of Geertz (1973) to help illustrate the relationship between work cultures and work identity. Geertz argues that people create for themselves a cultural identity and ideology which governs their behaviours and interactions within an organisation, since human actions can mean many different things and one needs to understand this in the context of the work setting. Tangherlini's (2000) work provides an explanation as to why storytelling appears prevalent within the paramedic profession, as he postulates that paramedics potentially become exposed to hostile and challenging situations and environments. These sometimes unpredictable situations can foster a relationship between storytelling and folklore, which Tangherlini alludes to the day-to-day rhythms of the work and their environment. By demystifying the concept of storytelling and folklore, we were reminded of Schein (2004) to draw together a collection of beliefs, values, and behaviours which go some way to help understand the relationship between storytelling and culture. The distinctive characteristics of certain organisations and institutions, where individuals have certain basic assumptions and ratify membership into a group. We believe this means that various nuances and subculture within the ambulance workforce reveal a discrete storytelling which is prevalent amongst individual paramedics whilst in the confines of the ambulance or ambulance station.

It would be remiss of us not to address the term 'black humour', or 'dark humour', 'gallows humour', in the context of paramedic language. It is a form of humour sometimes used by emergency personnel as a relief mechanism after dealing with traumatic situations, as also seen in the work of Christopher (2015). We wanted to assure ourselves that the 'storytelling' which I experienced in the workplace whilst collecting fieldnotes is not necessarily a form of dark humour used by the emergency services; instead, it was a different kind of humour! Scott (2007: 350) claims paramedics and police officers use a form of humour after witnessing horrific sights or when faced with incidents such as mutilated bodies. Several examples existed which contained examples of how humour helped in everyday practice, which she concludes 'authenticates the value of humour as a stress reducing mechanism and is a normalizing characteristic of emergency care culture'. Rosenberg

(1991) found that dealing with the physical exhaustion, emotional stresses, and at times challenging and dangerous situations, whilst responding rapidly to life-or-death situations, exposes individuals to high levels of personal anxiety. Humour can generate a feeling of personal accomplishment amongst emergency workers. McCreaddie and Wiggin's (2008) review of the literature associated with death and humour identified the use of humour as both challenging and revealing, particularly regarding self-deprecating humour. Scott (2007) advocates that this style of humour lies with people's values and the culture of the working environment. Despite Scott's explanation of emergency service personnel using dark humour as a coping mechanism, Metz (1981) and Corman (2016) provide examples, given here, which illustrate a type of behaviour that at times is somewhat bizarre.

> There seems to be a widespread agreement amongst them (EMTs) about how patients should be classified and about how the various classifications should be treated. In other words, the EMTs stereotype the patients and pass these attitudes along to trainees.
>
> (Metz, 1981: 113)

Whilst Corman recalls how:

> Jake goes on to explain how the call might impact his initial reaction to the call; if the call was an Echo (this is the call code indicating a critical incident), he might 'get excited'; however, if it was an Alpha call, (this is the call code indicating a non-critical incident) he thinks to himself, 'This [call] might suck'.
>
> Corman (2016: 34)

In comparison, the dark humour which Scott (2007) states is an essential coping mechanism for paramedics' day-to-day work as they become hardened to the sights they get to see. Corman (2017: 29) claims that 'they see things that are unfamiliar in everyday settings and interact with individuals who are in a backstage mode, whose defences are down, whose normal politeness has been shattered by crisis'. He found multiple professional identities are a consequence of the paramedics' role and the environment in which they work. Tangherlini's (2000) work is quite clear that the storytelling he identifies is not always dark (black) humour, but a form of storytelling which is steeped within the traditional working practices and traditions (banter) of the ambulance service and paramedic profession. Student paramedics' behaviour may be somewhat different when alone or with colleagues in the ambulance or the ambulance station, to that experienced in the classroom at university, which Lave and Wenger's (1991) work suggests is because students want to fit-in to the accepted norms of the working environment.

In this section, we have illustrated how literature on the use of paramedic storytelling has been explored, along with its influence and impact on the student paramedics' professional identity and working practices. The work of Geertz (1973) helps to contextualise cultural identities, and Tangherlini's (2000) work around folklore offers some understanding of storytelling. How and when paramedic storytelling occurs is sporadic and situational in the clinical practice setting. The next section of the chapter explores the concept of pedagogy and communities of practice (Lave & Wenger, 1991), which seeks to understand and establish how this concept forms part of the enculturation of student paramedics in their clinical practice setting.

## 3.7 Pedagogy and community of practice

There is a need to recognise and demonstrate that situational learning enables the application of knowledge depicted within the practice setting. Benner's (2015: 3) work on nurses helps explain this, as she suggests the 'signature pedagogy in nursing is designing experimental learning', as Lave and Wenger's (1991) seminal work positions learning in the practice setting as situated learning. This would mean the practice setting provides the platform for learning which is not necessarily the learning that is prescribed for the clinical setting. Becker et al. (1961) found trainees were often drawn into the working environment as they strived to complete their fresher's year, accepting poor working conditions and long working hours to achieve what was expected of them. Work-readiness of student paramedics may not necessarily be evident in the clinical placement setting, as paramedic students form part of a traditional workforce, taking on the established ways of working, such as undertaking minimal basic patient assessment and examination rather than the in-depth detailed assessment procedures taught at university. Willis et al. (2010) describe how the university community is a very different community from that experienced by students in the workplace. As Lave and Wenger (1991) also imply, the social setting forms a prominent part of the learners' community and formulates a dimension of social practice viewed as situated activity. Greenland (1977) suggests the curriculum becomes adopted as the practice setting exposes students to the nuances and traditions set within it. It is 'how things are done around here', rather than following the formal structured curriculum delivered at universities, whilst Benner's (2015) work considers the theories taught to the students in the classroom to that of the workplace. Lipsky's (2010) work implies that housing officers would pick and choose their clients based on ease, such as non-confrontational and quick wins, as opposed to lengthy complex cases. This is despite a formal selection policy and procedure which front-line housing staff were required to follow.

Palmer (1989), Metz (1981), and Corman (2017) found the traditional working practices of paramedics remained consistent throughout their individual studies, and Becker et al. (1961) provide an example of the demands placed on medical students within the authoritarian autocratic faculty.

A faculty member had done something the students resented very much, something that emphasised his power over them. I (Becker) sat and listened to a discussion of what they could do about this. One of the students said, 'One thing you have to understand is that most of us here will put up with just about anything if we really have to in order to get through. We spent too much time getting this far to start being crusaders about something like that. Whether you like it or not, we have to put up with it and we do'.

(Becker et al., 1961: 281)

Unwin et al.'s (2007) work contextualises the nature of pedagogy within the workplace setting, referring to the symbolic relationship between workplace learning and operational demands, whilst Fuller et al. (2011) highlight a complex relationship between learning and workplace, as both have competing demands and outcomes. This means that multiple modes of learning can have commonly occurring consequences for students. As suggested by Hafferty and O'Donnell (2014), these forms of pedagogy, whether by choice or coercion, can significantly influence student learning.

To understand the impact this can have on student paramedics, Willis et al. (2010) draw on the work of Benner (1984) to pose two arguments. Firstly, the Australian paramedic industry's expectations of an experienced practitioner do not necessarily reflect educational theory, and secondly the degree of knowledge and skills required to move beyond the novice stage originates from literature associated with sociology, law, ethics, psychology, and communication. This can indicate that the traditional in-house ambulance training model, familiar to both the UK and Australian ambulance services, is not sufficient to reflect the supporting sciences of sociology.

Willis et al. (2010) suggest the introduction of degree-level education leading to registration provides an opportunity to address these issues. This is significant, as developments in paramedic education become more educationally (university) based, and there is an expectation by the regulatory and professional bodies that this will drive change within the paramedic profession. We would argue, however, this has yet to be fully achieved, as students go into the workplace setting with a set of competencies in which to perform mechanistic practical skills, such as inserting a breathing tube into a patient's mouth or inserting a needle into the patient's vein. Yet the higher-level cognitive knowledge and social awareness required for the role of paramedics remain somewhat vague and absent, as the more traditional behaviours and practices drive the student learning. To address these issues, Willis et al. (2010) also argue that an educated reflexive and advanced practitioner with the growth of knowledge and understanding within the social sciences, which may be difficult to teach in the classroom setting, is required. Benner (1984) helps illustrate how nurses develop in clinical practice, suggesting:

The heart of the difficulty that the novice faces is the inability to use discretionary judgment. Since novices have no experience with the situation they face, they must use these context-free rules to guide their task performance. But following rules legislates against successful task performance because no rule can tell a novice which tasks are most relevant in a real situation or when an exception to the rule is in order.

(Benner, 1984: 128)

The sociological interpretation of pedagogy in practice, rather than skills acquisition alone, is decisive and can inform an understanding of the practice environment. The pedagogy which occurs because of the hidden curriculum, as Flamholtz and Randle (2011) believe, is significant and dependent upon the political, institutional, and social landscape in which students learn. In short, Flamholtz and Randle (2011) argue students possess a desire to form part of their workplace community, which Lave and Wenger (1991), Lipsky (2010), and Corman (2016) also note. Metz (1981) highlights the social solidarity of crews (communities) when unrealistic demands were placed on them from various sources, such as workload, shift patterns, reduced breaks, and downtime. Students are drawn into a form of community of practice which is based on a recognised traditional, established workplace community, which 'becomes the property of a kind of community created over time by the sustained pursuit of a shared enterprise' Wenger (1998: 45). Communities are formed from a shared purpose over a period, like paramedic students spending blocks of time in the workplace. Students become forged within a shared purpose as they become drawn into a particular community.

Members of these communities are formed by joining in common activities. This, as Wenger (1998) suggests, leads to either formal or informal communities being formed and stems from their mutual engagement in these activities. Pedagogy in practice remains fluid, tacit, and unstructured. Specific examples are woven throughout Chapter 5 to help elicit pedagogical behaviour of students. Connections are drawn between the practice setting and pedagogy. A dissonance exists between what is taught in the formal setting of the university and that in the practice setting.

The theoretical knowledge taught in university can enable student paramedics to rationalise and identify best practice. However, these practices are stifled and confused as students become inevitably caught up in a chaotic working environment. Consequently, tension and anxiety exist as students go into the clinical practice setting (Jones et al., 2010) unsure of their roles and responsibilities. In the next section of the chapter, we explore the literature to offer further explanation of why these tensions exist.

## 3.8 Tension

Wallis's (2009) work illustrates that a number of tensions exist between generations of nurses in the workplace as nurses of different decades work alongside each other. She argues that 'each generation holds different values which differs from others in the way they make sense of the world, and in what they expect from work' (Wallis, 2009: 62), whilst Putnam et al. (2014) believe tension in the context of the workplace possesses an overarching dilemma in implementing workplace flexibility, suggesting friction exists between the flexibility to work autonomously, with that of a rigid, controlling environment. This can also be seen in the work of Givati et al. (2018).

Considering the aforementioned discussion, the work of Sarros et al. (2002) was reviewed and it was found that tensions existed in their work on a bureaucratic, quasi-military style, US Eastern seaboard fire department, suggesting the style of leadership was a significant factor in this, as also seen in the studies of McCann et al. (2013) and Wankhade and Mackway-Jones (2015). Metz (1981) expresses the often taken-for-granted assumption that the work of EMTs and paramedics offers variety in the workplace. For example, Metz highlights how experienced EMTs/paramedics bracket certain incidents (jobs), such as calls involving minor injuries or trivial ailments, false alarms, and regular callers. The perceived inappropriateness of these calls causes low morale and tension between crews, as both students and experienced paramedics find these tensions cause unhappiness and dissatisfaction after working long hours, often without official breaks. Other influences include the time of day or night, nearing the completion of the shift, and calls early in the shifts (whilst the crew are checking their equipment and ambulance), and these all add to the tensions associated with the work of paramedics. An example here taken from our early fieldnotes helps illustrate this:

> I was riding out on an early shift with Charlie the student and Jim the paramedic. It was early morning (07–00 to 19–00) day shift. Whilst we were checking the ambulance equipment, stocking the paramedic drugs and checking the road worthiness of the vehicle (Ambulance), and at the same time having a cup of morning tea. A call was received from ambulance control at (07–01) for a male with head pains. The time of origin of the call (when the 999 call was first received by ambulance control was 05.30am), one and half hours prior to the call being despatched to us. Both Charlie and Jim were fuming at such an outrageous position to be in. We did not get back to station that day till 19–20.
>
> Taken from my fieldnotes (05/05/2014).

We postulate that there remains rigid managerial influence over ambulance work. Managerial control is exercised over crews, which includes electronic positioning location monitors (data-tracking devices) in the rig or truck (ambulance), which McCann et al. (2013) suggest causes additional tension amongst crews, as they witnessed direct control over crew staff (both paramedics and students). For example, they found managers physically hurrying crews out of hospitals in an attempt to exercise explicit and direct control over their working environment. They recall the lack of direction witnessed by one of the researchers during a particularly busy period of the day, as ambulance managers put pressure on paramedics to leave hospitals where they were waiting to hand over patients in order to get them back into commission and available for additional calls (McCann et al., 2013). Crew staff (paramedics and students) develop and implement their own style of working practices, which Lipsky (2010) explains is a form of survival within the workplace. Paramedics and students display a constant vigilance (lookout) for ambulance officers (managers), as any unnecessary downtime (unable to attend a call) is frowned upon by managers. This can occur at hospitals whilst crews create a little downtime or at the scene of incidents and back on station. The desire to experience freedom from direct supervision within the ambulance service is not new, as patient handover at hospitals along with the necessary cleaning of ambulances and completing of documentation that follows were often being neglected due to managerial pressure, which Givati et al. (2018), Wankhade and Mackway-Jones (2015), and McCann et al. (2013) conclude are conflictual restrictions that are present in ambulance services.

Like authors such as Bass and Riggio (2010), Judge and Piccolo (2004), and Avolio and Bass (2002), we suggest that as a result of deconstructing the institutionalisation of the ambulance organisation, a less bureaucratic management regime, which normalises and orientates the workforce to a more encompassing organisation, could be a more effective model of management. Swain (2019), however, urges caution here, suggesting that workers are familiar now with leaders and managers talking nonsense about leadership and employee autonomy. Swain (2019) makes a valid contribution here, concluding that this type of rhetoric is often used by managers to get their own way as ambulance services continue to function and operate as quasi-military style organisations, something which Sarros et al. (2002) have already identified and impacts significantly on the operation of the ambulance service.

In this section, literature pertaining to tensions associated with the institutionalisation of the ambulance service has been discussed. We highlight this as it serves to illustrate the subtle, often hidden forms of behaviour and working customs entrenched within ambulance work, which forms part of the wider makeup of the hidden curriculum and subculture. This contributes to shaping and influencing student enculturation of the practice environment. We summarise this section in the following with key points which emerged from the literature.

The literature implies that the impact of these tensions on the behaviour and workplace subculture of paramedic socialisation is important and can, in part, be summarised by Schein's (1985) model of organisational culture along with the behaviours and intricacies within the day-to-day working of paramedics and students. Using Schein's three-layer approach to culture, it is easy to see how different expectations are formed. For example, artefacts – the observable aspect of unconscious beliefs (responding to emergency calls). Espoused beliefs, values, and behavioural patterns – how the philosophy of the organisation operate, the vision and values of the ambulance service. Thirdly, assumptions – the embedded, taken-for-granted behaviours which are usually unconscious beliefs, such as the working practices within the organisation. McCann et al. (2013) illustrate how ambulance services operate as a quasi-military style fashion, whilst Metz (1981) and Mannon (1992) highlight the tensions created by the perceived mundane nature of the emergency calls which EMTs and paramedics attend. These are sources of frustration and tension between students and paramedics, which aggravates the tensions already experienced by crews. In the next section of the chapter, we explore how these experiences result in the enculturation of student paramedics in the workplace.

## 3.9 Enculturation

Reviewing the literature on enculturation reminded us of the affiliation with socialisation, so for the purpose of clarity we recap on the definition of the two terms to help focus our search. Gibson and Brightwell (2006) believe enculturation draws on established and accepted norms and values of a particular culture or society, where accepted members fulfil the functions and roles of the group. Kottak (2010: 23) describes enculturation as 'the process whereby individuals establish a context of boundaries and accepted behaviour that dictates what is acceptable and not acceptable within the framework of that society'. McPherson and Brown (1988: 267) define socialisation as 'the process whereby individuals learn skills, traits, values, attitudes, norms, and knowledge associated with the performance of present or anticipated social roles'.

Now that we had reminded ourselves of enculturation, the work of Choy and Delahaye (2011) was reviewed as they found students contextualised the formal taught elements of study within the sociocultural and functional environment of the workplace, suggesting students become enculturated into the workplace, before even experiencing it, whilst Willis et al. (2010) suggest graduates were not ready for the experience of clinical placements, as the relationship between work experience, institutionalisation, and professional identity is interwoven and is a consequence of an entrenched subculture and subsequent hidden curriculum.

Working practices influence the students' experience and learning environment, thereby enculturating the student into the traditional ways of working. This gives rise to a working environment which Brewer and Whiteside (2012) depict as an unfavourable, adverse, and often hostile way of working, whereupon unprofessional and unscrupulous practices can occur, such as bullying, sexism, racism, homophobia, and in some instances criminal behaviour, which may be prevalent within the day-to-day work of paramedics and student paramedics.

Lewis (2017: 7) reports the alleged misconduct at one NHS ambulance service trust, revealing a 'culture of bullying, harassment and alleged sexual predation at an ambulance trust that managers failed to address, leaving employees bereft of both confidence and direction'. Lewis's findings reveal a behaviour far removed from the formal process expected of managers. Subsequently, contradictory definitions, terminological and conceptual confusion can result, as the relationship between what happens in the practice environment, to that expected by the university is, and remains, polarised. This poses confusion and uncertainty for students as they enter the ambulance workplace.

Kramsch (1999) highlights the importance of recognising an individual's difficulty in abandoning already constructed cultural demeanour, behaviours, and values, when trying to customise to a new culture. Students are drawn into an unexpected, unintentional, unwarranted, and unhelpful practices when they attend clinical placements, as Corman (2017) found deep entrenched ways of working existed within the ambulance service, which is further supported by McCann et al.'s (2013) work with the UK inner-city NHS ambulance service trust. The enculturation of student paramedics enables them to function as members of a particular group or community. Its influences, amongst other things, include behaviours, expectations, rituals, symbols, and moral values, which students share with peers and newcomers and leads to a continuous cycle of enculturation:

A type of culture which forms a pattern of thought, emotions and behaviours which are learnt, not necessarily innate or inter-connected or shared within a group. Instead, it characterises each group, to what their relationships are with the environment and people.
(Hofstede & Bond, 1984: 417–433)

Tuohy et al. (2008) remark that culture itself is not static nor a single entity, rather there are multiple facets which change as one evolves through different environments and interactions.

In this section, the literature associated with the enculturation of paramedics has been reviewed. This comprises of a subculture which inadvertently produces a hidden curriculum. This hidden curriculum impacts and impinges on student learning and their subsequent enculturation into a formidable, established, and traditional culture, which leads to a form of pedagogy not experienced in university or envisaged by the students.

In the last section of the chapter, we summarise the interpretation of the literature whilst exploring the conceptual framework for this study. This provides an underpinning theoretical context, drawn out of the literature, and helps illustrate how and why paramedic students become enculturated into the traditional working ways and customs of the ambulance service.

### 3.9.1 Overview of the chapter

This chapter has reviewed both national and international literature pertaining to paramedic culture to encapsulate, compare, and contrast the various models of student paramedic enculturation. It was also necessary to explore how tension existed between individuals, with managers and crews, with students and paramedics, and with each other. We also explored similarities between the various types of ambulance cultures, such as the culture depicting paramedics as lifesaving heroes, as opposed to the expectations of the ambulance organisation, with that of the day-to-day working subculture which students become exposed to.

In order to explore, examine, and interpret the findings associated with the concepts of subculture, hidden curriculum, and pedagogy, evidence integral to these concepts has been discussed. In understanding these concepts, the work draws together developments of the paramedic profession both within and outside the UK to help contextualise the paramedic landscape.

The extent to which student paramedics' learning is influenced by pedagogy within the classroom setting has been shown to be limited. Whilst literature pertaining to pedagogy in practice provides meaning and context to this research, associated literature relating to social integration, behaviour, tension, and work experience has been discussed to help provide further context. Various sections of seminal works have been used, which directly relate to paramedic practice, whilst other seminal work complements and supports the wider body of knowledge which includes other professions such as the fire service, nursing, medical students, police officers, and housing officers. These are drawn from the prevailing literature to help provide support and agency to this study. Both of us, along with the participants of the study, have been influenced by this work. Our personal engagement has been compelling and significant in highlighting the issues raised by this research. The issues identified highlight significant expectations and potential differences in paramedic students' learning and learning environment which ultimately impacts on their professional values and pedagogic understanding. Based on this, the question then is to what extent students are drawn into the traditional taken-for-granted ways of working in the clinical practice environment of paramedic practice and what is the impact on their learning?

The methodology used to explore these concepts for this study is key to our findings, therefore we believe insight and understanding into why an ethnographic approach was adopted is an important component of our research and one which we believe will be helpful to share with the reader. Therefore, the next section looks at the research approach, whilst illustrating the methods used in our data collection.

## References

Agnew, R. & Kaufman, M. J. (2010) *Anomie, Strain and Subcultural Theories of Crime: The Library of Essays in Theoretical Criminology*. New York: Routledge.

Alsubaic, M. A. (2015) 'Hidden curriculum as one of current issue of curriculum', *Journal of Education and Practice*, 6(33).

Anyon, J. (1981) 'Social class and school knowledge', *Curriculum Inquiry*, 11(1), pp. 3–42.

Aultman, L. P., Williams-Johnson, M. R. & Schutz, P. A. (2009) 'Boundary dilemmas in teacher–student relationships: Struggling with "the line" ', *Teaching and Teacher Education*, 25(5), pp. 636–646.

Avolio, B. J. & Bass, B. M. (Eds.). (2002) *Developing Potential Across a Full Range of Leadership: Cases on Transactional and Transformational Leadership*. Mahwah, NJ/London: Lawrence Erlbaum Associates.

Ball, L. (2005) 'Setting the science for the paramedic in primary care', *Emergency Medical Journal*, pp. 896–900.

Bass, B. M. & Riggio, R. E. (2010) 'The transformational model of leadership', *Leading Organizations: Perspectives for a New Era*, 2, pp. 76–86.

Becker, H. (1963) *Outsiders: Studies in the Sociology of Deviance*. New York: The Free Press.

Becker, H., Geer, B., Hughes, C. E. & Strauss, L. A. (1961) *Boys in White*. New Brunswick, NJ: Transaction Books.

Bell, A. (2010) 'The subculture concept: A genealogy', in S. G. Shoham, P. Knepper & M. Kett (Eds.), *International Handbook of Criminology*. Boca Raton, FL: CRC Press.

Benner, P. (1984) *From Novice to Expert: Excellence and Power in Clinical Nursing Practice*. English – 1 January 1984. London: Pearson. ISBN 10: 020100299X ISB N 13: 9780201002997.

Benner, P. (2015) 'Curricular and pedagogical implications for the Carnegie study, educating nurses: A call for radical transformation', *Asian Nursing Research*, p. 3.

Blackman, S. J. (2014) 'Subculture theory: An historical and contemporary assessment of the concept for understanding deviance', *Journal of Deviant Behaviour*, 35(6). http://dx.doi.org/10.1080/01639625.2013.859049

Bourdieu, P. (1990) *In Other Words: Essays Towards a Reflexive Sociology*. Stanford, CA: Stanford University Press.

Bray, M. (2017) 'Schooling and its supplements: Changing global patterns and implications for comparative education', *Comparative Education Review*, 61(3), pp. 469–491.

Brewer, G. & Whiteside, E. (2012) 'Workplace bullying and stress within the prison service', *Journal of Aggression, Conflict and Peace Research*, 4(2), pp. 76–85.

Brewer, J. D. (2000) *Ethnography: Understanding Social Research*. Berkshire/New York: Mc Graw – Hill Education.

Burford, B. (2012) 'Group processes in medical education: Learning from social identity theory', *Medical Education*, 46(2), pp. 143–152.

Burford, B., Morrow, G., Rothwell, C., Carter, M. & Illing, J. (2014) 'Group processes in medical education: Learning from social identity theory', *Medical Educational*, 48(4), pp. 361–375.

Burt, C. (1925) *The Sub-Normal School Child: The Young Delinquent*. London: University of London Press Ltd.

Campeau, A. G. (2008) 'The space-control theory of paramedic scene-management', *Symbolic Interaction*, 31(3), pp. 285–302.

Care Quality Commission. (2015) https://www.cqc.org.uk/sites/default/files/2016 0721_annualreport_2015-16.pdf

Carlson, E., Pilhammar, E. & Wann-Hansson, C. (2010) ' "This is nursing": Nursing roles as mediated by precepting nurses during clinical practice', *Nurse Education Today*, 30(8), pp. 763–767.

Choy, S. & Delahaye, B. (2011) 'Partnerships between universities and workplaces: Some challenges for work-integrated learning', *Studies in Continuing Education*, 33(2), pp. 157–172.

Christopher, S. (2015) 'An introduction to black humour as a coping mechanism for student paramedics', *Journal of Paramedic Practice*, 7(12), pp. 610–617.

Clinard, M. (1974) *Sociology of Deviant Behaviour*, 4th ed. New York, NY: Rinehart and Winston.

College of Paramedic's Curriculum Guidance Framework. (2019) https://collegeof paramedics.co.uk/?gclid=Cj0KCQjwqs6lBhCxARIsAG8YcDhZ5NQeSilXkhny3r CZar2RjVxkoY--4ecNyLV8wg-3THvxjpoD0R0aAqrfEALw_wcB

Corman, K. M. (2016) 'Street medicine – Assessment work strategies of paramedics on the front lines of emergency health services', *Journal of Contemporary Ethnography*, 46(5), pp. 600–623.

Corman, K. M. (2017) *Paramedics on and off the Streets-Emergency Medical Services in the Age of Technological Governance*. Toronto/Buffalo/London: University of Toronto Press.

Coster, S., Norman, I., Murrells, T., Kitchen, S., Meerabeau, E., Sooboodoo, E. & d'Avray, L. (2008) 'Interprofessional attitudes amongst undergraduate students in the health professions: A longitudinal questionnaire survey', *International Journal of Nursing Studies*, 45(11), pp. 1667–1681.

Cottingham, H. A., Suchman, L. A., Litzelman, K. D., Frankel, M. R., Mossbarger, L. D., Williamson, R. P., Baldwin Jr, C. D. & Inui, S. T. (2008) 'Enhancing the informal curriculum of a medical school: A case study in organisational culture change', *Journal of General Internal Medicine*, 23, pp. 715–722.

Cowell, R. N. (1972) *The Hidden Curriculum: A Theoretical Framework and a Pilot Study* (EdD thesis, Harvard Graduate School of Education).

Cox, A. (2005) 'What are communities of practice? A comparative review of four seminal works', *Journal of Information Science*, pp. 527–540.

Delamont, S. (2008) *How to do Education Ethnography*. Edited by G. Walford. London: The Tufnell Press.

Department of Health. (2008) *Pre-Registration Education and Funding for Paramedics: Guidance for SHAs, PCTs and Ambulance Services*. London. http://www.dh.gov. uk/en/Publicationsandstatistics/Publications/PublicationsPolicyAndGuidance/ DH_085225.

Devenish, A. S. (2014) 'Experiences in becoming a paramedic: A qualitative study examining the university qualified paramedics', *Creative Education*, 7(6), pp. 786–801.

Doja, A., Bould, M. D., Clarkin, C., Eady, K., Sutherland, S. & Writer, H. (2016) 'The hidden and informal curriculum across the continuum of training: A cross-sectional qualitative study', *Medical Teacher*, 38(4), pp. 410–418.

Donaghy, J. (2010) 'Equipping the student for the workplace changes in paramedic education', *Journal of Paramedic Practice*, 2(11), pp. 524–528.

Dreeben, R. (1968) Cited in Kentli, F. D. (2009) 'Comparison of hidden curriculum theories', *European Journal of Educational Studies*, 1(2), pp. 83–88.

Boychuck Duchscher, J. E. & Cowin, S. L. (2004) 'The experience of marginalisation in new nursing Graduates', *Nursing Outlook*, 52, pp. 289–296.

Evetts, J. (2003) 'The sociological analysis of professionalism: Occupational change in the modern world', *International Sociology*, 18(2), pp. 395–415. SAGE Publishing.

Flamholtz, E. & Randle, Y. (2011) *Corporate Culture: The Ultimate Strategic Asset*. Stanford, CA: Stanford University Press.

Fuller, A. & Unwin, L. (2011) 'Workplace learning and the organization', *The SAGE Handbook of Workplace Learning*, pp. 46–59.

Geertz, C. (1973) *The Interpretation of Cultures.* New York, NY: Basic Books.

Gibson, B. & Brightwell, R. (2006) *The Developments in Paramedical Science and the Implications of National and International Accreditation and Registration in Alliance with Ambulance Authorities.* EDU-COM International Conference. Edith Cowan University. Australia.

Ginsberg, S., Regehr, G., Hatala, R., McNaughton, N., Frohna, A., Hodges, B., Lingard, L. & Stern, S. (2000) 'Context, conflict and resolution: A new conceptual framework for evaluating professionalism', *Academic Medicine*, 75(10), pp. 6–11.

Giroux, A. H. (2001) *Theory and Resistance in Education: Towards a Pedagogy for the Opposition.* Westport, CT/London: Greenwood Publishing Group.

Givati, A., Markham, C. & Street, K. (2018) 'The bargaining of professionalism in emergency care practice: NHS paramedics and higher education', *Advances in Health Science Education*, 23, p. 353.

Greenland, J. (1977) *An Investigation into Aspects of the Hidden Curriculum* (Doctoral dissertation, University of Oxford).

Greenwood, E. (1984) *Self-Actualization for Nurses: Attributes of a Profession.* Rockville, MD: Aspen Systems Corp, pp. 13–26.

Hafferty, F. W. (1998) 'Beyond curriculum reform: Confronting medicine's hidden curriculum', *Academic Medicine*, 73(4), pp. 403–407.

Hafferty, F. W. & O'Donnell, J. F. (2014) *The Hidden in Curriculum in Health Professional Education*, 1st ed. Hanover, New Hampshire: Dartmouth College Press.

Hammersley, M. & Atkinson, P. (1993) *Ethnography – Principles in Practice,* 2nd ed. New York: Routledge.

Health and Care Professions Council. (2023) *Standards of Proficiency (Paramedics),* 3rd ed. London. https://www.hcpc-uk.org/globalassets/standards/standards-of-proficiency/reviewing/paramedics---new-standards.pdf

Henderson, S. (2002) 'Factors impacting on nurses' transference of theoretical knowledge of holistic care into clinical practice', *Nurse Education in Practice*, 2(4), pp. 244–250.

Hofstede, G. & Bond, M. H. (1984) 'Hofstede's culture dimensions: An independent validation using Rokeach's value survey', *Journal of Cross-Cultural Psychology*, 15(4), pp. 417–433. https://doi.org/10.1177/0022002184015004003

Hundert, E. M. (1996) Cited in D'eon, M., Lear, N., Turner, M. & Jones, C. (2007) 'Perils of the hidden curriculum revisited', *Medical Teacher*, 29(4), pp. 295–296.

Jackson, P. W. (1968) *Life in Classrooms.* New York, NY: Holt, Reinhart & Winston.

Jones, A., Slater, J. & Griffiths, P. (2010) 'The first-year experiences of paramedic students in higher education. A mixed evaluation', in *Health Science and Practice.* London: Higher Education Academy, p. 37.

Judge, T. A. & Piccolo, R. F. (2004) 'Transformational and transactional leadership: A meta-analytic test of their relative validity', *Journal of Applied Psychology*, 89(5), p. 755.

Kell, C. & Owen, G. (2008) 'Physiotherapy as a profession: Where are we now?' *International Journal of Therapy and Rehabilitation*, 15(4), pp. 158–164.

Kelly, A. V. (2006) *The Curriculum Theory and Practice*, 5th ed. London/Thousand Oaks/New Delhi: SAGE Publishing.

Kottak, C. P. (2010) *Window on Humanity a Concise Introduction to Anthropology,* 4th ed. New York, NY: McGraw-Hill.

Kramer, M. (1974) *Reality Shock: Why Nurses Leave Nursing.* St Louis: C.V. Mosby Company.

Kramsch, C. (1999) 'Cultural perspectives on language learning and teaching', cited in Knapp, K., Seidlhofer, B. & Widdowson, H.'s *Handbook of Foreign Language Communication and Learning*. Berlin/New York: Mouton de Gruyter.

Lave, J. & Wenger, E. (1991) *Situated Learning: Legitimate Peripheral Participation*. Cambridge/New York/Melbourne/Madrid/Cape Town/Singapore/Sao Paulo/Delhi: Cambridge University Press.

Lewis, D. (2017) *Workplace Culture at Southwestern Ambulance NHS Foundation Trust*. London: An Independent Report Commissioned by The South Western Ambulance Service NHS Foundation Trust in partnership with UNISON.

Lewis, E. O. (1933) 'Types of mental deficiency and their social significance', *Journal of Mental Science*, 79, pp. 298–305. https://doi.org/10.1192/bjp.79.325.298

Lipsky, M. (2010) *Street-Level Bureaucracy Dilemmas of the Individual in Public Services*. New York: Russel Sage Foundation.

Lovegrove, M. & Davis, J. (2013) *Paramedic Evidence-Based Education Project (PEEP). End of Study Report*. Buckinghamshire: Allied Health Solutions/Buckinghamshire New University.

Mackintosh, C. (2006) 'Caring: The socialisation of pre-registered student nurses: A longitudinal qualitative study', *International Journal of Nursing*, 43(8), pp. 953–962.

Madden, R. (2010) *Being Ethnographic: A Guide to the Theory and Practice of Ethnography*, 2nd ed. London/Thousand Oaks, CA/New Delhi/Singapore: SAGE Publishing.

Mannon, M. J. (1992) *Emergency Encounters – EMTs and Their Work*. Boston, MA: Jones and Bartlett.

Matheson, R. (2019) 'In pursuit of teaching excellence: Outward and visible signs of inward and invisible grace', *Teaching in Higher Education*, 25(8), pp. 909–925.

McCann, L. (2022) *The Paramedic at Work: A Sociology of a New Profession*. New York/Oxford: Oxford University Press.

McCann, L., Granter, E., Hyde, P. & Hassard, J. (2013) 'Still blue-collar after all these years? An ethnography of the professionalisation of emergency work', *Journal of Management Studies*, 50(5), pp. 750–774.

McPherson & Brown (1988) Cited in Brustad, R. J. (1992) 'Integrating socialization influences into the study of children's motivation in sport', *Journal of Sport and Exercise Psychology*, 14(1), pp. 59–77.

Mead, G. H. (1936) *Movement of Thought in the Nineteenth Century*. Edited by M. Moore. Chicago/London: University of Chicago Press.

Metz, L. D. (1981) *Running Hot-Structure and Stress in Ambulance Work*, 1st ed. Edited by L. D. Metz. Cambridge, MA: Abt Books.

Mulder, H., ter Braak, E., Carrie, H., Chen & Olle ten Cate. (2019) 'Addressing the hidden curriculum in the clinical workplace: A practical tool for trainees and faculty', *Medical Teacher*, 41(1), pp. 36–43. https://doi.org/10.1080/01421 59X.2018.1436760

Nelson, L. (1997) Cited in Griffiths, E. (2015) 'The search and rescue helicopter paramedic: An emerging role', *Journal of Paramedic Practice*, 7(8).

Newton, A. (2012) 'The ambulance service: The past, present and future (part 1)', *Journal of Paramedic Practice*, 4(5), p. 8.

Nurok, M. & Henckes, N. (2009) 'Between professional values and the social valuation of patients: The fluttering economy of pre-hospital emergency work', *Social Science & Medicine*, 63(3).

O'Donnell, J. F. (2014) *Introduction: The Hidden Curriculum – A Focus on Learning and Closing the Gap, Medical Teacher*. Hanover: Health Professional Education, Dartmouth College Press.

O'Meara, P. (2011) 'So how can we frame our identity?', *Journal of Paramedic Practice*. paramedicpractice.com.

O'Reilly, K. (2009) *Key Concepts in Ethnography*. London: SAGE Publishing.

Palmer, E. (1983) ' "Trauma Junkie" and street work: Occupational behaviour of paramedics and emergency medical technicians', *Journal of Contemporary Ethnography, Urban Life,* (2), pp. 162–183.

Palmer, E. (1989) 'Paramedic performance', *Sociological Spectrum,* 9, pp. 211–225.

Parsons, T. (1942) 'Age and sex in the social structure of the United States', *American Sociological Review,* (7), pp. 604–616.

Pratt, M. G., Rockmann, K. W. & Kaufmann, J. B. (2006) 'Constructing professional identity: The role of work and identity learning cycles in the customization of identity among medical residents', *Academy of Management Journal,* 49(2), pp. 235–262.

Putnam, L. L., Myers, K. K. & Gailliard, B. M. (2014) 'Examining the tensions in workplace flexibility and exploring options for new directions', *Human Relations,* 67(4), pp. 413–440.

Reynolds, J. (2007) 'Discourse of inter-professionalism', *The British Journal of Social Work,* 37(3), pp. 441–457.

Reynolds, L. (2004) 'Is prehospital care really a profession', *Journal of Emergency Primary Health Care,* 2.

Rosenberg, L. (1991) 'A qualitative investigation of the use of humour by emergency personnel as a strategy for coping with stress', *Journal of Emergency Nursing,* 17, 197–203.

Sarros, J. C., Tanewski, G. A., Winter, R. P., Santora, J. C. & Densten, I. L. (2002) 'Work alienation and organisational leadership', *British Journal of Management,* 13, pp. 285–304.

Schein, H. E. (1985) *Organisational Culture and Leadership,* 2nd ed. San Francisco, CA: Jossey-Bay.

Schein, H. E. (2004) *Organizational Culture and Leadership,* 3rd ed. San Francisco, CA: Jossey-Bay.

Scott, T. (2007) 'Expression of humour by emergency personnel involved in sudden death work', *Mortality,* 12(4), pp. 350–364.

Stenhouse, L. (1975) 'Defining the Curriculum Problem', *Cambridge Journal of Education,* 5(2), pp. 104–108.

Stevenson, Elliot & Jones. (Eds.). (2002) *Concise Oxford English Dictionary,* 2nd ed rev. Oxford University Press.

Strauss, C. & Quinn, N. (1997) *A Cognitive Theory of Cultural Meaning* (No. 9). Cambridge/Victoria/Madrid/Cape Town: Cambridge University Press.

Swain, R. D. (2019) 'Leadership lessons through the lens of historical military leaders: A pedagogical approach to teaching leadership theories and concepts in a Masters of Public Administration course', *Teaching Public Administration,* 37(2), pp. 234–252.

Tangherlini, R. T. (2000) 'Heroes and lies: Storytelling tactics among paramedics', *The Folklore Society. Routledge Journals,* 111(1), pp. 43–66.

Tangherlini, T. R. (1998) *Talking Trauma-Paramedics and Their Stories*. Jackson, MS: University Press of Mississippi.

Taylor, S. J. & Wendland, C. (2014) *The Hidden Curriculum in Medicine's "Culture of No Culture": The Hidden Curriculum in Health Professional Education*. London: Dartmouth, pp. 53–62.

Thornton, S. (1995) *Club Culture, Music, Media and Subculture Capital*. Cambridge/Oxford: Polity.

Tindall, B. A. (1975) 'Ethnography and the hidden curriculum in sport', *Behavioural and Social Science Teacher*, 55(2), pp. 164–170.

Tuohy, D., McCarthy, J. & Cassidy, L. (2008) 'Educational needs of nurses when nursing people of a different culture in Ireland', *International Nursing – Wiley Online Library*, 55(2), pp. 164–170.

University of Hertfordshire. (2020) https://www.whatuni.com/degrees/paramedic-science-bsc-hons/university-of-hertfordshire/cd/54930514/1040/

Unwin, L., Felstead, A., Fuller, A., Bishop, D., Lee, T., Jewson, N. & Butler, P. (2007) 'Looking inside the Russian doll: The interconnections between context, learning and pedagogy in the workplace', *Pedagogy, Culture & Society*, 15(3), pp. 333–348.

Vallance, E. (1986) 'A second look at conflicting conceptions of curriculum', *Theory into Practice*, 25(1), pp. 24–30.

van der Gaag, A. & Donaghy, J. (2013) 'Paramedics and professionalism: Looking back and looking forwards', *Journal of Paramedic Practice*. Mark Allen Group, 5(1), pp. 8–10.

van Maanen, J. (2011) *Tales of the Field: On Writing Ethnography*, 2nd ed. Chicago/London: The University of Chicago.

Wallis, L. (2009) 'Born to be different: Today's nurses span four generations, and this can lead to tension in the workplace', *Nursing Standard*, 23(33), pp. 62–64.

Wankhade, P. (2015) 'Different cultures of management and their relationships with organisational performance: Evidence from the UK ambulance service', *Public Money & Management*, pp. 381–388.

Wankhade, P. & Mackway-Jones, K. (2015) *Understanding the Management of Ambulance Services Ambulance Services: Leadership and Management Perspectives*. Cham/Heidelberg/New York/Dordrecht/London: Springer.

Wenger, E. (1998) *Communities of Practice Learning, Meaning and Identity*. Cambridge/New York/Victoria/Madrid/Cape Town: Cambridge University Press.

Wilkinson, A., Hislop, D. & Coupland, C. (2016) 'The changing world of professions and professional workers', in *Perspectives on Contemporary Professional Work*. Cheltenham/Northampton, MA: Edward Elgar Publishing.

Williams, B. & Webb, V. (2015) 'A national study of paramedic and nursing students' readiness for interprofessional learning (IPL): Results from nine universities', *Nurse Education Today*, 35(9), pp. e31-e37.

Willis, E., Williams, B., Brightwell, R., O'Meara, P. & Pointon, T. (2010) 'Road-ready paramedics and the supporting sciences curriculum', *Focus on Health Professional Education: A Multi-Disciplinary Journal*, 11(2), pp. 1–13.

Woollard, M. (2009) 'Professionalism: Professionalism in UK paramedic practice', *Journal of Emergency Primary Health Care (JEPHC)*, 7.

Young, M. (1995) 'Black humour: Making light of death', *Policing and Society*, 5, pp. 151–167.

# 4 Methods of enquiry

## 4.1 Introduction

In this chapter, the research methodology is laid out. It starts by discussing the research paradigm and goes on to describe the methods used in the study, which comprise of ethnographic observations accounting for most of the data and a small number of interviews to disclose student perspectives and the lived experiences revealing processes of enculturation. Finally, the chapter concludes how the chosen methodology influences and shapes the study. The next section of this chapter discusses the research paradigm. Table 4.1 provides an illustration to help illuminate the various stages of the research process.

## 4.2 Research paradigm

Hawker (2006: 494) defines a paradigm as 'a pattern or model of something'. A constructivist paradigm consists of the learner having previous experience and knowledge which is usually determined by their cultural and social environment. Seifert et al. (2008: 33–37) believe 'learning is therefore done by students constructing knowledge out of their experiences'. This is illustrated by Kuhn (1996: 10) who believes that 'a paradigm implies a set of concepts and practices that define a scientific discipline at any particular period'. Exploring a notion such as culture within the paramedic workplace required a methodology which enabled us to tease out detailed intricacies and nuances, which are often unseen by those who may be outside the research-specific subject, as illustrated by Madden (2017: 20) who suggests that 'many characterisations of ethnography will stress the emic or insider perspective over the etic outsider perspective to understand the folk or native insider point of view'. We were mindful of Madden's words and never lost sight of my own perspective of being both an insider and, at times, an outsider researcher, along with the driving question as to why student paramedics appear to change their behaviour when they attend the clinical practice setting. Qualitative research allows the exploration necessary to study the experiences and voices of a group or population, sometimes making it possible to hear silenced voices, as

DOI: 10.4324/9781032721408-4

*Table 4.1* Overview of research project

| | |
|---|---|
| Research Title | An examination of |
| | University Paramedic students' Enculturation into the Ambulance Service |
| Study | Explored student paramedics' understanding and experience of their practice placements. |
| | Focusing on their integration with their more experienced paramedic colleagues. |
| Methods | Ethnography |
| | Revealed the real-life, day-to-day events which students experience in their clinical work placements. |
| Ethics | Institutional, ambulance service and NHS ethics clearance |
| Pilot Study | Tested fieldnote data collection and interview schedule with students. |
| Paradigm | Constructivist Paradigm |
| Main Study | Explore students' experiences. |
| | Institution, National Institute of Health Research (NIHR), NHS Ambulance Service Trust Ethics |
| Design | Ethnography: |
| | Data was obtained over 18 months, using observational fieldnotes, interviews, and reflexivity. |

| Methodology Methods | Qualitative | Fieldnotes | Interviews | Sample interviews based on accounts of fieldnotes (n = 8) |
|---|---|---|---|---|

| | |
|---|---|
| Pilot Study | Explored social integration into the community of practice and that of the paramedic |
| Main Study | **Total Sample:** Key participants n = 8. Other participating participants n = 30 |
| | **Time Period:** Between 2013 and 2014, 18-month period. |
| | **Area:** Predominantly inner-city Metropolitan, along with leafy suburban rural areas |
| | **Research Tool:** Ethnographic field notes supported with semi-structured interviews. |
| | **Qualitative Analysis:** thematic coding by hand, supported with electronic supporting software. |
| Pre-defined Key Areas | Professional Identity, Institutionalisation, Work experience. |
| | Pedagogy woven throughout the three themes. Embedded within communities of Practice. |
| Emergent Sub Themes | Traditional ways of working, bullying, meal breaks, stress, uniforms, late finishes, management support, working colleagues, training, ambulance control, vehicles, management spies, whistle blowing, workload, university curriculum, superheroes, Pre-judgement, patients, racism, sexism. |
| | How students became enculturated into the community of practice (Ambulance Service) |

seen in the work of Cresswell (2007). Creswell refers to observational studies, in particular hearing the silent voice. Drawing on observational studies in the latter part of the investigation enabled us to tease out a detailed understanding of the subject matter as well as the voices of the paramedic students.

The paradigm was identified by the research aim, which was to explore student paramedics' enculturation into the ambulance service. We were interested in the process of how, and why, student paramedics appear to engage with certain values and ways of working. Of particular interest is the socialisation which appears to take place between the established traditional workforce and new recruits; the central aim of ethnography is, as Spradley (1979: 3) points out, 'to understand another way of life from the native point of view'.

Individual students perceive their experience differently, as they interpret or make sense of the situation within the context of their points of reference. In turn, the researchers' individuality inevitably contextualises and affects the research. Crotty and Crotty (2004) refer to this as multiple constructed realities. Therefore, the texts produced during observations are, as Mann (1992: 273) describes, 'never an objective record of what happened, rather, an expression and interpretation'. Consequently, an interpretivist paradigm allows the researcher to elicit, engage, and connect with participants, uncovering aspects of the individuals, such as their feelings, thoughts, and behaviours, along with the individuals' expectations. Within this process, certain interests, assumptions, and the researcher's perspectives may be different to the issues being researched. This can potentially influence the research and must be identified and acknowledged. However, caution is required as Madden (2017: 25) suggests that 'The influences of subjectivity on ethnography and the lack of control over field settings are the sorts of conditions that are mentioned when people make a claim that the ethnography is not scientific or reliable'. We were always mindful and never lost sight of the fact that the relationship between the researcher and participants is pertinent and essential to the ethnography. Both have a different construction of social realities, making the method of data collection a key component in drawing out rich insights into the study's context (Brewer, 2000). In using an interpretive position, we attempt to reflect on the realities of the findings (Denzin & Lincoln, 2002), produce judgements about the data and translate this to the book. By choosing this paradigm, several assumptions were imposed, namely that the application of theoretical classroom knowledge into the clinical practice setting is complex, made up of conscious and subconscious processes which are contextually constrained. This allowed for the opportunity to reveal and illuminate the nuances, intricacies, and subtleties of the paramedic practice setting. The next section of this chapter considers ethnography in more depth.

## 4.3 Ethnographic principles

Guba believes a set of guiding beliefs form the infrastructure of the research paradigm, which Guba (1989: 18) expresses as an inquiry which asks: 'What is the nature of knowledge or reality (ontology)? what is the relationship between the researcher and knowledge (epistemology)? and how the inquirer should go about finding out knowledge (methodology)?'.

We wanted an approach which explored the interaction between the often knowledgeable but inexperienced neophyte paramedic students and the authoritative stance of the experienced paramedics. Givati et al. (2018) highlight that to facilitate this, an insider's (emic) view of the realities of the workplace, as opposed to an outsider's (etic) understanding, was identified (Pike, 1967). According to Madden (2017: 6), 'ethnography is ultimately a story that is backed up by reliable qualitative data and the authority that comes from active ethnographic engagement'. This is further supported by Spradley (1979: 5) who believes that 'ethnography is concerned with illustrating meanings of actions and events of people, through observation and interviewing key informants', whilst O'Reilly (2009: 3) claims that 'ethnography is a theory, or set of ideas, about research that rests on a number of fundamental criteria', that it is iterative-inductive research, and that it evolves in design through the study. However, ethnography is not without critics who may view this kind of data collection as subversive and non-scientific. For example, Hammersley (2018) found critics argue that ethnographers can fail to examine the processes through which the phenomena studied have been constituted, suggesting there is an absence of rigour due to unexplicated common-sense knowledge. In our view, this criticism is subjective which only becomes problematic if due processes and procedures have not been followed regarding the ethnography, for example following good practice, such as accurate note taking, recording events and situations as they are seen through the researcher's lens, and respecting participants' anonymity. Draper (2015) believes these all contribute to ethnographic principles.

John's background as the UK-registered paramedic provides considerable expertise and experience in identifying the subtleties and complexities this research captures. The ethnography is used to explore and gather insight into the realities of the participants' experiential viewpoints based on details of what occurred, which Brewer's (2000) work helps to reveal, what is said (Koch, 1996), between the lines (Kvale, 1996), and silences (van Maanen, 2011). The individuals' perspective of their experience is considered in relation to the context in which it is positioned. This illuminates the participants' cultural and social experiences. John's reflexive interpretation of the participants' experiences could then be taken back to the participants in follow-up interviews. This revealed an exploratory lens based on shared experiences which helped to uncover participants' reality as it was experienced and interpreted by them. Hammersley and Atkinson (2006) express the importance of ethnographic enquiry in uncovering the emerging issues which they believe can be found by the ethnographer as:

> Researchers participating, overtly or covertly, in people's daily lives for an extended period of time, watching what happens, listening to what is said, and/or asking questions through informal and formal interviews,

collecting documents and artefacts – in fact, gathering whatever data are available to throw light on the issues that are the emerging focus of inquiry.

(Hammersley & Atkinson, 2006: 3)

Geertz (1973) found that participants act and behave differently and voice their opinions openly, depending on the relationship with the ethnographer. The participant's voice is influenced by the ethnographer's insider or outsider status. Notwithstanding the researcher's emic or etic stance, participants often express their rationale and meaning about individuals, their environment, and the way of illustrating this to the researcher. Walford (2008) believes that:

Ethnography is the art and science of describing a group or culture. The description may be of a small group in an exotic land or a classroom in middle-class suburbia. The task is to interview relevant people, review records, weigh the credibility of one person's opinion against another and look for ties to special interests and organisations.

(Walford, 2008: 272)

Recognising Walford's (2008) description, the need to identify the ties to any specific community or group which occurred in the practice setting was acknowledged. Creswell (2007) helps identify how to investigate such a phenomenon, as he believes qualitative research supports exploration, especially the need to identify a group or community, illuminate specific irregularities which can then be measured, or to listen to silent voices. Creswell speaks of the 'silent voice', referring to the intricacies of nonverbal communication and body language. Observations will allow the opportunity to elicit various trends which may be explicit in a participant observation. Schwandt (2007: 96) reminds us that 'Ethnography is a particular kind of qualitative inquiry distinguishable from case study research, descriptive studies and naturalistic inquiry by the fact that it is the process and product of describing and interpreting cultural behaviour'. John's focus was to unpick and understand the subculture which we are arguing exists. Therefore, the need to understand how a subculture may impact on the students' learning and enculturation into the paramedic profession and the subsequent hidden curriculum which gives rise to it is important.

Considering the aforementioned discussion, drawing on an emic perspective, enabled a more nuanced insider interpretation and understanding of the experiences and shared meaning of participants (van Maanen, 2011) as they react to, and within, a culture. This provides a clear description of social meaning. The ethnographic principle of cultural interpretation locates the researcher as an integral part of the research process, as also seen in the work of Madden (2017), O'Reilly (2009), Brewer (2000), Walford (2008), and van Maanen (2011). Ethnographers engage with their research, exploring the perspectives of participants and assimilating the researcher's own views to help aid the research. Denzin and Lincoln (2008) describe interpretivism as mutual patterns of impressions encapsulated in the participants' experience. O'Reilly (2009: 122) suggests interpretivism is to 'understand shared meanings, cultures, and individual motives that lead to action'. These are articulated by the researcher through a rich, explicit depiction of the individual, societal, and cultural aspect of the situation being investigated. Savin-Baden (2004) believes a reflexive researcher provides the reader with insight and understanding of the relationship between the research study and the researcher's position within the study. This enables the researcher's background to be disclosed, decisions made, and the strategies formed for the readers to see.

The next section of the chapter looks at the data collection methods used.

## 4.4 Methods

To ascertain which data collection tools to use, we firstly considered the conceptual framework employed for this study, as the purpose of data collection is to elicit information and understanding from participants (Brewer, 2000). Although our work eventually ended up as an ethnography, we initially explored Kelly's (1955) Personal Construct Psychology's (PCP) Reparatory Grid (RG) as part of a small-scale study. This introduced John to his research journey and provided an indication that, after their first clinical practice placement, the expectations of the paramedic students, about the workplace, appeared to have changed. This early work provided the foundation from which to draw comparisons, between first-year university students going into the workplace and those returning from the workplace environment. This illustrated the fact that some cultural influences which were embedded within the structure of the ambulance service were affecting students. For instance, John found student perceptions altered, after workplace exposure, compared with their perceptions prior to the workplace; this puzzled us, and we wondered what was going on.

Data generated in this process illustrated the need for further investigation to determine the phenomenon of student enculturation. Furthermore, it became evident from the initial dataset that an in-depth understanding of the complexities may best be achieved from an insider's perspective of the phenomenon using field observations as an insider to the profession. Consequently, the concept of utilising an ethnographic approach to establish why this phenomenon appeared to be prevalent within the paramedic profession was undertaken, therefore John as a paramedic practitioner and principal researcher carried out the data collection. Adler and Adler (1987), Lipsky (2010), Palmer (1989), and Metz (1981) draw on the richness and in-depth analyses of ethnography in examining the inner workings of emergency service personnel. It also became clear, through reflecting on the initial experiments with PCP, that exploring culture within the workplace can require more than one method within the researchers' armament if one is to gain a deep and meaningful experience from the data collection (Denzin, 2017).

## 4.5 What method to employ

The use of an ethnographic approach meant we could identify an appropriate data collection tool. Both interviews and focus groups have a long traditional standing in the data collection of qualitative research methods (Cresswell, 2007). These were supplementary methods to our fieldnotes. However, Patton (2002) believes participants may amend or change their behaviour and react differently in focus groups or interviews, as these methods can sometimes provide socially suitable answers. By this Patton suggests interviews and focus groups can lead students to provide answers which they believe the researcher wants to hear. Our aim was to understand how and why university paramedic students become socialised into a very different workplace culture, to that cultivated at university. To do this, I (John) needed to hear, see, and experience what was really going on in the workplace setting, to hear the voices and probe questions in the attempt to gain insight into the students' perspectives of the workplace environment. I acknowledged that some students and experienced paramedics may know me, both as an academic and/ or paramedic practitioner, and therefore may not wish to voice their opinion or express their views openly to me in interviews and focus groups, which may have led to participants acting differently or expressing opinions which they may believe I wanted to hear and see from them and limiting confession. Although there is a risk of the researcher's observations affecting behaviour, I become immersed in their day-to-day work. I remembered Atkinson et al.'s (2007) work suggesting that ethnography limits and restricts these possibilities, as students become immersed in the day-to-day working practices. Following the critique of the literature, along with our desire to really understand what was happening in the workplace, we referred to Becker et al.'s (1961: 133) work, who believed that 'the most complete form of sociological datum, after all, is the form in which the participant observer gathers it; this rich data gives more information about the event under study than data gathered by any other sociological method'. O'Reilly (2009) concludes:

> Being with people (or more precisely, being ethnographic with people), in their time and space, in all their strangeness and in their mundane and quotidian flow, is still one of the most valued ways to build a qualitative understanding of the particularities and generalities of the human condition.
>
> (O'Reilly, 2009: 143)

Here, we are not suggesting that other forms of enquiry are not valued and valid. They are more than adequate to provide a different lens in which to illustrate enculturation of student paramedics into the workplace setting.

However, we are indicating how, for us, participant observation was an appropriate, yet challenging, method with which to explore, uncover, identify, and illustrate the intricacies and behaviours often unseen and unknown to those outside the practice setting. Diamond (2008) provides an ethnographic account of patients in long-term care facilities in the USA, and Rankin and Campbell (2006) give an ethnographic explanation of nursing. These studies depict the use of ethnography to help illustrate the social interactions of people in the healthcare setting and provide reassurance to us that our approach is both workable and valid. These two studies are particularly helpful as the subjects being explored were patients and nurses who found themselves in challenging and at times distressful situations. These findings are similar with that of paramedics who often work in hostile and challenging situations and environments. The seminal work of authors such as Corman (2017), McCann et al. (2013), Palmer (1983), and Metz (1981) helps to understand the complexity of the challenging working environments of paramedics' work, along with the cultural discourses which are displayed by those who work in the organisations. Metz's (1981) work is particularly helpful in providing an historical account and understanding of how the ambulance crew's behaviours, customs, and unwritten rules became a prominent feature in their day-to-day operational working practice. Madden's (2017) work expresses how ethnography synthesises the information gathered by the ethnographer by contextualising the fieldnotes (data), into a narrative, suitably structured as to illustrate the ethnographer's journey. Metz's study spanned a period of several years, two years employed as an emergency medical technician (EMT) in America working alongside other EMTs and paramedics, whilst undertaking an extensive ethnography as a researcher. His work affords recognition and provides authority and realism to this unique working environment. His study recognised the cultural meanings, institutional rules, and rituals of the EMTs and paramedics within a competitive socioeconomic backdrop of austerity. He determines and illuminates the human activities of this working environment (Metz, 1981) and galvanises the historical past with the 1980s, to provide a sociological perspective of ambulance culture. More recently, Corman's (2016) work on Canadian paramedics suggests the research often assumes an operational perspective rather than empirically exploring what paramedics do in their day-to-day work. Authors such as Creswell (2008), Brewer (2000), Walford (2008), van Maanen (1990), and Hammersley (1993) describe the richness and depth of thick description which is attributed to ethnography as a sociological form of enquiry.

Drawing on the work of Brewer (2000), I (John) generated my fieldnotes from the observational placements, audio-recordings, interviews, and the occasional report to help draw out meaning from the data and clarify my findings. Burgess (1985) suggests this overtly engages the researcher with the participants and their communities of practice, which Lave and Wenger

(1991) also identify. Burgess (1985) stresses the positive impact he believes insider researchers have, arguing they can achieve full participant status as someone who already belongs to the group being researched. Hammersley (1993), however, suggests there are no overwhelming advantages to being an insider or an outsider researcher. I kept in mind both Burgess's and Hammersley's advice and was very cognisant of the professional boundaries which I, and students, may experience in the day-to-day clinical practice environment. To address this, I, very early on in the data collection phase of the research, joined in with the banter and culture of the workplace. I tried to give an illusion of being a paramedic, being one of them, although I never lost sight of Walford's (2008) views, which highlight the danger of the insider researcher going 'native' arguing that this infers the researcher is trying to be the person he/she is researching, rather than as a researcher. Labaree (2002) argues that one can simultaneously be to some extent an insider and to some extent an outsider, of qualitative research, as the research may have elements of insiderness, along with outsiderness attached to it. I am a registered paramedic and was not trying to become native, instead I wanted to get a real appreciation for what I was seeing, hearing, experiencing, and recording. As suggested by Madden (2017), I was trying to make the familiar unfamiliar. Walford (2008) also points out that the position of insider/outsider research is endorsed by one's reflexivity. Kielmann's (2012) ethnography focuses on practitioners and their professional socialisation within healthcare as being reflexive. In undertaking this research, I had to balance the dichotomy of insider/outsider relationships. I became reflexive and reflected on the research and participants' relationship to help understand and position myself within the role of researcher.

Establishing the relationships between the researcher, student paramedic, and experienced paramedic became somewhat tested in the field. As seen in the work of Creswell (2008), research participants view the researcher through multiple lenses. I attended operational shifts both in ambulance uniform and, at times, non-uniform. When I attended operational shifts without my uniform, however, it appeared to cause some anxiety for both students and experienced staff. I continued to test this by wearing my ambulance uniform for many of the shifts, then occasionally I would arrive for the shift in my normal clothing, except for my protective footwear (steel toe-caped boots) and high-visibility fluorescent jacket, which is mandatory for riding out on ambulances. I thought of Burgess (1985) who believes a fundamental part of being an ethnographer is to become accustomed and accepted into the social context of the community being observed. Brewer (2000) suggests as an ethnographer it is essential to immerse oneself into a community to gain deeper insight of the intricacies and nuances which may not be so clearly obtained from literature or methods where information could be second-hand. Ethnography obtains insight into the participants' lives (O'Reilly, 2009), the customs, traditions, intricacies, and nuances of their day-to-day environment, which may not be attainable through a narrative discourse alone. Here the researcher has a relationship with the participants, the community activities, and the wider research environment. Extensive and elaborate notes are recorded of the experience. This enables the researcher to engage with the culture without imposing one's own social reality (Searle, 1995) on that culture (Walford, 2008). Craft and Jeffrey (2008: 141) propose that 'ethnographic research includes involvement, immersion and empathy on the one hand and distance, scientific appraisal and objectivity on the other'. I never lost sight of their view.

## 4.6 The research study

The study consisted of a number of paramedics from a traditional inner-city NHS ambulance service trust, many of which were long-serving members of staff who had trained as paramedics through the traditional in-house, Institute of Health Care and Development (IHCD) award a few years ago, before university paramedic degree programmes existed. In addition to the paramedics, eight university paramedic students offered their time to help in the study. Numerous other students became involved in the study along with other consenting paramedics as I came across staff and students at various locations, such as hospitals and ambulance stations and at times on scene of incidents. These participants knew of my data collection due to information circulated via the internal ambulance service network and by word of mouth. In addition, students from the university where I worked were aware of the research project. Consequently, I carried a supply of information sheets and consent forms which were circulated to participants to ensure I remained within the ethical boundaries of the research project. O'Reilly (2009: 63) suggests 'Ethical issues are best resolved via an ongoing reflexive dialog between the researcher and research participants within the field context'.

The eight student paramedics selected for the study were observed over a period of 12–18 months, often on 12-hour shifts, consisting of a student paramedic along with an experienced paramedic or newly qualified IHCD paramedic (NQP). Semi-structured interviews were used to support and supplement the observational fieldnotes, and the purpose of these interviews was to gain a deeper understanding and clarification of my observational findings (Brewer, 2000; Burgess, 1985). This helped to complement and contextualise the data and facilitate exploration of the student's own views of the phenomenon under investigation.

Table 4.2 provides an example of my time collecting data. The matrix identifies whether data was collected from students, newly qualified paramedics (NQPs), experienced paramedics, or other members of ambulance staff or emergency service personnel. This example gives an indication of when and where the data was collected, such as hospitals, on the scene of an incident, in the ambulance station, or in the ambulance vehicle, and highlights the total time accrued collecting fieldnotes (602 hours) and the total

*Table 4.2* Example of data collection matrix (2013–2014)

| Data Collection Method | Fieldnote Duration | Interview Duration | Student Pseudonyms Names | Paramedic/ EMT Pseudonyms Names | Other e.g. Firefighter, Nurse, Police officer, Pseudonyms Names | Location of data Collection |
|---|---|---|---|---|---|---|
| Fieldnotes | 12 Hour shift | N/A | Janet | Asher | Other Ambulance personnel | Ambulance Station |
| Fieldnotes | 12 Hour shift | N/A | Tony | Time | N/A | At the Hospital |
| Fieldnotes | 12 Hour Shift | N/A | Tom | Bill | N/A | Ambulance Station |
| N/A | N/A | 1 Hour | Jennie | N/A | N/A | At University |
| Fieldnotes | 12 Hour shift | N/A | James | Bruce | N/A | In the Ambulance |
| Fieldnotes & Interviews | 12 Hour shift | 1 Hour | Amy | Tina | Other Ambulance personnel | On-Scene |
| Fieldnotes | 10 Hour shift | N/A | N/A | N/A | N/A | In the Ambulance |
| Fieldnotes & Interviews | 8 Hour Shift | 45 Minutes | Ben | Joe | N/A | In the Ambulance |

number of interview hours (10 hours). Table 4.3 provides examples of short biographies of participants involved in the study. We have used pseudonyms to protect the individual identity of participants.

## 4.7 Study site

Clarification to undertake the research was sought from the university's research and ethics unit, the NHS ambulance service trust, where the study was going to be conducted, and the National Institute for Health Research (NIHR). This process proved to be complex and lengthy, before receiving permission required to access the study-sites.

We were mindful that the ambulance service was a type of regimented organisation which I recognised may take some time for approval. Brewer's (1991) ethnography of policing in Northern Ireland offers an understanding of the relationship between a structured authoritarian militaristic organisation, such as the Irish police authority, and the researcher. It was not plausible or realistic to proceed with my research study if negotiations between us and the organisation's gatekeeper(s) involved in the study were not established and agreed prior to data collection (Madden, 2017). There was close liaison with the ambulance service trust, for which we are personally grateful for the opportunity to start data collection, and we looked forward to involving participants in their daily working lives for an extended period of time.

*Table 4.3* Example of participants biographies

| Participants Name | Approximate Age | Gender | Ethnicity | Biographies |
|---|---|---|---|---|
| Ben | 18 | Male | White | 3rd year BSc Hons students + 150 hours clinical experience |
| Peter | 26 | Male | Mediterranean | 2nd year part-time Foundation degree student who is employed by the ambulance service |
| Paul | 58 | Male | White | An experienced paramedic with over 28 years ambulance service experience |
| Claire | 22 | Female | White | 3rd year BSc Hons students + 150 hours clinical experience |
| Tom | 20 | Male | White | 1st year part-time Foundation degree student who is employed by the ambulance service |
| Julian | 26 | Male | European | A Newley Qualified Paramedic (NQP) with 2 years operational experience |
| Jennie | 17 | Female | White | 2nd year BSc Hons student + 70 hours clinical experience |
| Julie | 20 | Female | White | 2nd year BSc Hons student + 70 hours clinical experience |
| Joe | 55 | Male | White | An experienced Paramedic with 21 years operational experience |
| Tim | 33 | Male | White | An experienced paramedic |
| Caroline | 17 | Female | White | 1st year BSc Hons student + 20 hours clinical experience |
| James | 17 | Male | White | 1st year BSc Hons student + 20 hours clinical experience |
| Mark | 22 | Male | European | A comparatively new paramedic training via the traditional IHCD training route |
| Lee | 32 | Male | Afro-Caribbean | 1st year part-time Foundation degree student who is employed by the ambulance service |
| Richard | 60 | Male | White | An experienced paramedic with over 20 years ambulance service experience |

I was keen to explore what was really happening to paramedic students in the workplace. I cite Hammersley and Atkinson as a reflection of my feelings and excitement of starting data collection: 'Watching what happens, listening to what is said, asking questions – in fact, collecting whatever data are available to throw light on the issues that are the focus of the research will contribute to the understanding' (Hammersley & Atkinson, 2006: 1).

Three specific ambulance complexes were identified for the research. Each complex comprised of two to three individual ambulance stations, which we are calling 'satellite' stations. This meant I could collect data from eight different ambulance stations, comprising of various working conditions and a mix of busy urban ambulance stations, along with some rural leafy suburban ambulance stations. It was important to encompass and investigate both urban and rural areas if we were to truly engage in forging the strange and the unknown elements of enquiry. van Maanen (2015: 44) is of the opinion that it is 'both dynamic and recursive but the encounter with the "foreign" or "unknown" or "strange" is the very essence of ethnography'. The ambulance stations selected also supported several university students in their clinical work placements from other universities. This was acknowledged early within the research process and identified as a risk as the site-specific ambulance locations could become saturated with students. Additional site-specific ambulance complexes had also been identified to reassure ourselves that sufficient site-specific stations were available. However, these additional facilities were not required as our concerns proved unfounded and participants in the study were accommodated within the eight original ambulance stations initially identified. This is where students had been allocated for their work placements. At times though, students were relocated to other ambulance stations at short notice due to the operational demands of the ambulance service. A number of these ambulance stations were some considerable distance away from where the student was initially meant to be attending. I too as the principal researcher sometimes had the unenviable task of chasing around a particular area trying to locate where students had been sent to work. Access to these ambulance stations were through gatekeepers, in this case the local ambulance station managers and local ambulance officers. Burgess (1983) highlights the importance of communication through which the researcher should exercise skill in building relationships and building rapport. Madden (2017: 52) believes that 'the ethnographic field represents part geographic location, part social and part mental construct, suggesting the conceptualisation of the interrogative boundary forms part of the ethnographic field of enquiry'.

Some local ambulance mangers became suspicious and sceptical of my purpose in their ambulance stations. To facilitate the manager's uncertainty and concerns, I carried copies of my research aims, along with the approval and consent documents, which I had previously received from the ambulance service, the NIHR, and the university. This helped to inform and reassure the ambulance managers (officers).

## 4.8 Participants

The selection of participants for the study was, in part, driven by the students' work rotas. Our thoughts were clear; we wanted to investigate the process of student enculturation in the workplace. To help illustrate and clarify the selection criteria, we provide some understanding of the process. I selected participants who were either employees of the ambulance service or paramedic degree students from the university, or a combination of both, as some students were studying a paramedic foundation degree programme. This meant that these students were also employed by the ambulance service trust on a short-term contract for a period of one year, as well as university students who attended university in blocks. The participants' shift patterns were challenging and raised several additional issues for me as the principal researcher. The day-to-day demands placed on me by fulltime employment in a large, busy university were challenging. I often conducted my observational fieldwork after a day's work at the university. I would leave work and attend late shifts or night shifts at nearby ambulance stations. I attended weekend shifts and took annual leave to attend additional shifts on ambulances. I raise this, not as a limitation of the study, but, as a consequence of data collection in the field of ethnography and a real understanding of the demands and challenges this brings. To quote van Maanen (2015: 41) 'Nothing much can prepare you for intensive fieldwork'.

## 4.9 Sample size and study duration

We took guidance from Patton (2002) and adopted purposeful sampling as the means of participant selection to the study. I selected students for their relevancy to the research and consent to study.

The students studying on the Bachelor of Science (BSc Hons) degree programme in Paramedic Science attended between two- and four-week practice placement blocks throughout the year. Students studying on the Foundation Degree programme attended clinical placement for one full year as employees of the ambulance service. These practice placements became the basis by which students become conditioned and cemented into the cultural and social aspects of the workplace environment. We drew on Lave and Wenger's (1991) work to help illustrate some similarity, as they refer to groups or communities, eventually having full legitimacy to contribute and engage within a profession.

To obtain the rich meaningful data, we initially struggled and pondered on the size and number of participating students. We eventually took comfort from Schwandt's (2007) work who suggests that the size of the sample depends on the study and the research questions and concepts under investigation. Hammersley's (2018) look at issues of adequacy of sample size in qualitative research is determined by several factors, including the phenomenon of data saturation. Hammersley's view suggested data saturation can become problematic. However, we also acknowledged that the data extrapolated from the students and experienced paramedics, along with secondary data, would produce a significant degree of data, suggesting generalisability of the data findings may be pertinent to other paramedic workgroups, along with academic institutions offering paramedic education programmes in the future. Brabbie (1989) suggests saturation of data in ethnographic fieldwork means that no additional data is found, and the ethnographer can develop themes from the categories.

All participants of the study were informed of the type of study being undertaken. This was conducted through the dissemination of information, such as email correspondence, posters, information leaflets, and flyers, throughout the ambulance service trust. Other dissemination methods included word of mouth and a detailed information letter which was issued to those participants who expressed an initial interest in participating in the study.

### 4.9.1 Ethics

It was imperative to our professional accountability and personal integrity that ethical approval was gained prior to carrying out any data collection. Madden (2017) illustrates the importance of gaining ethical approval by 'first, do no harm', whilst Higginbottom (2004: 4) talks of 'leaving ethical footprints which future researchers may follow, in the knowledge the research was conducted ethically'. Cohen (1981) believes the researcher should have a moral compass which ensures the reliability and validity of the research.

Informed consent was gained as an important and inseparable component of the research process which adds accountability and sensitivity to the work. Cresswell (2007) further suggests assigning aliases to participants, thereby protecting their privacy. Outlining the purpose and process of the research, along with participant anonymity, is an essential component of the researcher's role prior to data collection. Participants were advised that involvement in this study was entirely voluntary. Participants could withdraw from the study at any time, resulting in their data being destroyed. Assurance was also given that at no time would dialogue between the principal researcher and participants take place within the presence of any critically ill or injured patient if this would impede or disrupt the care provided to the patient. This was an important element to the study and one which was highlighted within the ethics application and subsequent approval of the study. It was essential that students, along with other participants of the study, such as the experienced paramedics, of whom students worked alongside, were able to consent to the research freely and informatively. This required participants to be fully informed of the study. This task proved challenging at times as individual (crew members) who may have initially been identified to work with the student for a particular shift, a task which was the responsibility of the ambulance resource centre, had sometimes been changed, swapped, or cancelled at short notice due to operational demands. This would result in other individual paramedics being drafted in at short notice as replacements. In these instances, I also carried with me an abridged résumé of the study which provided these paramedics with an outline of the study prior to the start of shift. In addition, all participants were provided with consent forms for both the pilot study and main study. Participants had the opportunity to ask questions about any aspect of the research. They were assured and guaranteed that any recordings and fieldnotes would remain in a secure and locked unit for the duration of the research. I was able to assure participants that their identity and university/employment organisation would be concealed. Cohen and Golan (2007) believe participant's rights, welfare, and dignity must be protected. Over the period I was collecting data, just one experienced paramedic refused to participate in the study. His/her actions were fully understood and appreciated, and I returned home instead of riding out and collecting data on the ambulance that day.

The interpretive nature of my research meant that the ethical aspects of the research emerged slowly, although some were identified early in the research process, and others appeared throughout the fieldwork and, as documented in the following, had aspects that went much deeper than formal procedures covered, such as understanding my role as researcher and practitioner should I need to assist with the treatment of a patient along with the ethical consequences. Madden (2017: 35) suggests that 'ethnography is a "whole body experience" and ethical commitment from the very outset, and through all phases of ethnographic research and writing is important'. We were also mindful that ethical commitment forms an integral and ongoing component of the research process. We wanted student paramedics, along with experienced paramedics and paramedic mentors, to participate in open and frank dialogue in quite detailed and, at times, emotive discussions around their perceptions of the day-to-day working environment. I was aware throughout the data collection that certain aspect of my fieldwork may be particularly sensitive to some participants. It was essential therefore that informed consent, along with a participant's autonomy and right to withdraw, be assured from the outset of the study.

Due to the unpredictable nature of paramedic work, interaction would sometimes occur whilst the student and paramedic were dealing with patients. Subsequently, patients were present during periods of the data collection, although they were not the primary focus of the study. Anonymity for the project was assured throughout the research process, and no individuals are identifiable within the research findings. Should any emotional or physical distress been caused to any participants either as a result of the research or from their day-to-day work, they would have been supported by the appropriate NHS ambulance service trust's counselling services and/or university counselling services.

As a registered paramedic, I was the principal research investigator in the field. I also have a duty of care. Prior to data collection, I recognised that there was a realistic prospect that occasions may arise whereby a patient's medical condition(s) or severity of an injury could become compromised if for some reason I decided not to intervene as a registered paramedic in the interest of patient safety. I grappled with the notion of the insider/outsider relationship in relation to this. Madden (2017) suggests insider/outsider relationships are not incompatible, rather they are simultaneously created and sustained as part of ethnographic fieldwork. The realistic potential of becoming involved, along with my ability to withdraw myself from the study as the researcher, should I be required to attend to a patient, could not be guaranteed. I took my strategy for managing and coping with any such eventuality from the HCPC Standards of Conduct, Performance and Ethics (2016) which states:

> You must take all reasonable steps to reduce the risk of harm to service users, carers and colleagues as far as possible'. And that you must not 'do anything, or allow someone else to do anything, which could put the health or safety of a service user, carer or colleague at unacceptable risk.
>
> (HCPC, 2016: 6.1 & 6.2)

The ethics approval application had to be realistic, timely, yet a pragmatic representation which recognised the possibility of allowing me the opportunity to gather data, whilst being mindful of my duty of care as a paramedic. Schwandt (2007: 89) refers to ethics as 'the justification of human actions, especially as those actions affect others'. On two occasions, whilst collecting data, I had to intervene as a paramedic. This first occurred whilst the crew and I were responding in the ambulance to a 999 emergency call for a road traffic collision (RTC). As we arrived on scene, I could see that several patients required medical attention, some of them urgently as they were in a critical condition. As we were the only ambulance crew on scene at that time, consisting of a paramedic, a student paramedic, and myself as a researcher, we quickly requested assistance via the ambulance radio transmitter to ambulance control, asking for urgent back-up. I recognised I had a duty of care and ceased being a researcher to take on the role of a paramedic. I put down my pen and notepad and assisted with the care and treatment of the patients. On the second occasion, I assisted an experienced (old-timer) paramedic with a clinical drug calculation as I became drawn into helping an elderly male who had collapsed and was in cardiac arrest. I again put my notepad in my pocket and assisted with the treatment and management of the patient. My notepad remained in my pocket for the duration of the patient care. Yet despite our best efforts, we were unsuccessful in resuscitating this patient.

### 4.9.2 *Pilot testing*

Initially a pilot study was undertaken to test the strategies and procedures. According to van Teijlingen and Hundley (2002: 33–36), 'pilot studies are a crucial element of good study design'. The pilot study allowed us to be reasonably assured that the practicalities of data collection, such as travelling, to and from the ambulance stations, resting between fulltime university work and data collection, on-site car parking facilities, public transport facilities to and from the data collection sites (ambulance stations), working around data collection, family life, and writing up findings, proved realistic. This also allowed us to test the quality of the data collection instruments, such as recording fieldnotes and my personal notes, as we sped through the busy inner-city traffic, undertaking one-to-one interviews, along with the quality of recordings. Brewer (2000) notes that pilot studies should be completed before the topic is pursued properly. Walford (2003: 76–77) helpfully illustrates this in his ethnography on elementary schools, when he states: 'He firstly conducted a pilot study in two elementary schools in a rural part of the prefecture, observing classes, interviewing teachers, and fine-tuning data collection instruments'.

I attended several ambulance shifts, known as ride-outs, as part of my pilot study. I recruited four students, along with four experienced paramedics, for the pilot study prior to the main ethnography. These eight (four student paramedics and four experienced paramedics) participants had been informed about the aims of the study along with their rights as participants in the study and the protection of their autonomy in the findings. Ambulance shifts were arranged so I was able to attend two night shifts on Friday and Saturday nights between the times of 19:00 to 07:00 hours, along with two day shifts, on alternative Saturdays and Sundays between the times of 07:00 to 19:00 hours. The shifts were repeated to ensure I had a spread of initial primary data from the eight individual participants over a period of ten weeks (eight 12-hour shifts in total). By undertaking these shifts over a period of weekends, I was able to continue with my fulltime employment at university throughout the week (Monday to Friday). Lynn et al. (2018) found field-based research offers an exceptional opportunity for in-depth research. However, the requirements of carrying out research away from home create challenges which are not necessarily always fully understood.

### 4.9.3 Initial stage of data collection

At the initial stage of the study, there were some unanticipated issues. We had to be assured the fieldnotes were recorded accurately, a true representation of what I had seen through the researcher's lens (Hammersley, 2018), at the end of each shift. I would use short follow-up interviews to check and verify my data in the form of fieldnotes, rather than presenting a narrative of events. This process proved difficult, however, as both the experienced paramedics and students were keen to leave work at the end of an often very busy 12-hour shift. I have to say, I too was also keen to get home on occasions.

We were aware that a component of my data collection strategy had been halted. We set in place plans to deal with this untoward eventuality. The majority of the shifts in the pilot study were extremely busy, unrelenting, and non-stop working. It was clear from the pilot study that the idea of reviewing and checking my fieldnotes with participants after each shift would be challenging and not a realistic proposition. We found a way around this problem as I decided to clarify any uncertainty in my fieldnotes at the time of writing them, or at the earliest opportunity within the field. This appeared to work well. I also used this strategy in the pilot study when in the presence of patients. I thought it unreasonable and rude to take extensive fieldnotes at the patient's side, although I needed to capture the dialogue which took place between both the paramedic and student whilst they were with the patient. This data was important as it had the potential to highlight any prejudices and nuances which manifested between the student and paramedic whilst treating the patient. Therein glimpses were gained that may not have neces- sarily been evident to me if I had left the room. In these circumstances my fieldnotes were documented as soon as practically possible after the patient had been cared for because I was mindful not to disrupt or delay any clinical intervention that may have been required for the patients. I also used any downtime (between calls) to write up my notes, such as free time when no emergency calls were pending. I used my fieldnotes to structure the interview process, to elicit data, and to reiterate my understanding of events and clarify situations. I was again reminded of Madden (2017: 71) who suggests 'the eth- nographer should express cultural ignorance when undertaking ethnographic interviews with participants, by using expressions such as: "I never knew that", or I didn't realise that you were so'. This keeps the information flowing as a form of corrective knowledge as participants clarify misunderstandings or perceived ignorance of the researcher. This system appeared to work well and proved helpful in understanding and clarifying certain aspects of the findings. These reflections I considered invaluable in helping to understand how and why students became enculturated into the working environment of the ambulance service (Schon. 1983). O'Reilly's (2009) assertions that pilot studies are useful in identifying issues that may arise from fieldwork were welcomed. Therefore, pre-testing of the observational data collection and interview process helped refine and clarify the fieldnotes into a more orderly and comprehensive set of records and reflections. For example, they provided additional insight and clarification of what I was experiencing. Conflicting views and understanding of events became visible as students and paramedics helped to clarify the plausibility of my interpretation.

The preliminary data source of the ethnography was fieldnotes which provided a snapshot of the day-to-day nuances and intricacies of the para- medics' working practices. It was pertinent that the qualitative nature of the ethnography revealed the representativeness of participants' interaction and socialisation into the working environment. Firstly, I was aware that, due to my status as a paramedic and academic, students and practitioners may have been reluctant to work and act as they would if I was absent. Secondly, despite emphasising that they should express themselves as they normally would on a day-to-day working shift, I was aware that this could be chal- lenging and may take some time. Thirdly, participants may have feared being perceived as negative with negative consequences for their programme of study or employment. Gagliardi et al. (2009) suggest participants may be unwilling to fully engage due to repercussions, or influence on professional relationships which remain after the research has been concluded. To address this early within the data (pilot) collection exercise, as an insider researcher, I used my experience as a paramedic to fit-in to the relationships. I was mindful of Abdullah's (1992: 8) observation about the use of 'verbal seduction, to encourage participants to share and depict their experiences'. I used a language which suited the workplace environment, the intricacies, nuances, colloquialisms, and behaviours, commonly used throughout the shift. We provide an example here to help illustrate how the day-to-day language was used within ambulance service interactions.

---

Whilst I was in the watch room I said to Robert, the Paramedic that I was going into the yard (ambulance station) to help Tony, the student with checking the truck (ambulance) and to just let us know if a job comes in down the line. By this I refer to us receiving an emergency call from ambulance control. Robert gave a smile as to approve my stance!
Taken from my fieldnotes (18/07/2013).

---

I was, to some degree, a native to the culture being studied. Madden (2017) suggests being native in an investigation can be problematic, as the researcher can become a form of 'participant' rather than researcher. I was mindful of this as I found participants became more relaxed and comfortable to have me around them and increasingly animated in both their dialogue and openness. The pilot study helped refine the data collection process, along with my position within the field, as I started to become drawn away from the native stance. It enabled an initial practice of ethnographic field studies. I felt more comfortable that the tool was not just adequate but also appropriate in eliciting the information and insights we wanted to experience from this study in relation to the research question.

### 4.9.4 Personal and analytical notes

I recorded in my fieldnotes various events, behaviours, language, dialogue, intricacies, nuances, subtleties, and discriminations which took place between students, paramedics, mentors, and patients, along with other key individuals. It is the ethnographer's duty to 'watch what happens, listen to what is said, ask questions, and produce a richly written account' (O'Reilly, 2009: 3). In addition to the accounts recorded in my fieldnotes, van Maanen (1990) believes ideas, impressions, and memories of the experiences are recorded in a journal to help decisions or create an audit trail which would assist during interpretation of data. Madden (2017: 139) believes ethnographers 'go to a great deal of effort to record good fieldnotes; they experiment with various styles, formats and jottings whilst wrestling with the reactivity notebooks can sometimes cause', an observation also supported by Atkinson et al. (2007).

During my time in the field collecting data, I drew on reflection to under-stand and critique my thoughts and views of what I had seen, heard, and experienced. I used my reflexive values to help relay my position as an emic, although at times etic, researcher. I allowed time whilst I collected my field-notes to record my insights and emerging ideas of what I was experiencing through a reflexive lens. At times I was exhausted, so it became challenging to accurately record my thoughts and feelings as footnotes to my data. Where this was the case, I wrote short notes and symbols which would help me revisit these later to prompt my memory. I was aware that my interpretation of what I had seen and recorded may have multiple meanings in different situations which I was keen to clarify with participants using short interviews (van Maanen, 2011) as and when I could.

### 4.9.5 Data analyses and management

Analysis of the research consisted of a process of constructing data by exam-ining various trends, themes, and the connection between them. The study used a qualitative ethnographic approach to address the enculturation of a group of university paramedic students into the clinical workplace of an ambulance service.

The ethnography enabled me to facilitate in-depth observational data through the collection of fieldnotes. I reflected on my actions during my observations in the field. This helped me to construct shared meanings to assist me in making sense of the observations which I had recorded in my fieldnotes and galvanised the perspectives of the participants. I described how my influence on the research process helped draw out situational meaning which contributed to some contextual understanding of student paramedic enculturation. O'Reilly (2009) suggests that ethnographic principles of cul-tural interpretation, which underpins this research, is not a prescribed set of methods, but rather a process which recognises the complexity of the human experience and human behaviour.

We drew on my personal insight, on literature from previous studies of the paramedic profession, both nationally and internationally. I immerged myself in the data, recapping and reflecting on my notes. By adopting a reflexive stance, I was able to draw on my experience to help understand and examine the data. We took van Maanen's (2011) guidance, figuring out realist tales, to authentically represent the cultural depiction of the text of the fieldnotes. We familiarised ourselves with the data, thoroughly examining and inter-preting my fieldnotes to dwell on the situation I had recorded. The data was separated into three main work-streams, consisting of, firstly, data recorded as fieldnotes, which comprised most of the data, secondly data recorded from face-to-face interviews with participants, which helped clarify certain obser-vations, and thirdly my reflections. We were drawn to O'Reilly's (2009: 70) interpretation of fieldnotes which is more focused on 'observations, jottings, full notes, intellectual ideas, and emotional reflections'. To enable meaning to be extracted from the raw fieldnotes, the researcher moves back and forth between data and recordings. My data produced three main streams, consisting of work experience, institutionalisation, and professional identity. At the centre lies pedagogy. The data was then sub-divided into themes then more manageable reasoned thematic trends, which van Maanen (1990) suggests is a process of isolating the thematic statements into detailed understanding and experiences of participants. Each element of data was coded as various themes and trends emerged together. Coffey and Atkinson (1996) suggest that coding separates and divides the data into manageable sections which can then be formulated into different interpretations. Key words, phrases, situations, and experiences of the data were searched to help elicit and capture the context of the ethnography. This process was undertaken by hand and recorded into text from the original hand-written fieldnotes and transcriptions of audio recordings. Once these had been transcribed onto electronic data using supporting software, it allowed us to draw various themes together more succinctly, alter or amend the data into various components, and scrutinise the findings more clearly. We took LeCompte and Schensul's (1999: 2) guidance that 'ethnographers create ethnography in a sometimes tedious and often exhilarating two-step process of analyses of raw data and interpretation of analysed data'. The fieldnotes were structured to record significant concepts emerging from the data, such as ideas, interpretive thoughts, views, and areas requiring clarification. I also attached my notes obtained from the face-to-face interviews between students and paramedics. This helped complement and enhance the data. We ensured that I was able to identify which dataset corresponded with each component of the data collection method. We attached a section whereby I was able to record my personal thoughts and reactions annotated in my fieldnotes. Once the initial data was separated into more manageable sections, we were then able to draw out detailed themes. This process began by initially selecting events, statements, situations, language, environments, with the public or without the public in private, also other work colleagues and students, nursing and medical staff, and lastly patients. These statements were then highlighted so key words, phrases, people, or situations were colour-coded and were categorised. This process continued as we refined the data drawn out from the fieldnotes and interviews. Patton (2002) believes that this is an essential process for qualitative data. Table 4.4 provides some early categorisation of my data to help illustrate the processes. This helped us to make sense of my fieldnotes and interviews.

We wanted to illustrate shared and conflicting phenomena of what we were investigating, to extrapolate meaning from what the data was telling us. Consequently, we re-categorised elements of data and re-ordered it into clusters before tabulating and sieving the data between themes, which van Maanen (1990) suggests in his work. Once the data had been rearranged into similar categories, two months were spent revisiting, re-ordering, and re-shaping the data that were similar or different. We were obtaining meaning

*Table 4.4* Example of early data categorisation clusters

| *Colour categorisation of data clusters* | *Example of my fieldnote and interview dataset* |
|---|---|
| Work Experience | Tony, the student, gave a number of examples of events where there had been problems. Each event has a student paramedic at the heart of the incident. We spoke about 'dangerous Jim', a paramedic, whom I had worked with just a few weeks previously with another student whilst collecting data. Tony referred to dangerous Jim as 'fucking Coco the clown'. I asked why Coco the clown? Jim answered, 'he is a fucking menace and difficult to work with. He's just a clown'. |
| Professional Identity | Although (Roy) is a newly qualified paramedic (NQP), he is very territorial and overrides students or constantly appears to question the decisions with patients whilst the student is questioning the patient at the time. Rebecca, the student, appeared to stop talking, not challenge Roy, but rather accepts his authority as an NQP and just works under his instructions. This did not appear to be mentorship, but a form of power. |
| Work Experience | As soon as I started the shift it was apparent that there were tensions between the crew. When I had the opportunity, I spoke with the student (Tom), I asked him why such hostility between them both (him and his crewmate) the paramedic (Bill). Tom threw his eyes to the back of his head and said, 'John, he is a knob, Bill doesn't want to be here and he takes it out on us (students) although he is okay with his old stooges' (I took this to mean the experienced old hands) 'and he seems okay with you John, but that's because you are a visitor'. |
| Work Experience | I could see the student (Chris) struggling to cope with the enormity of dealing with a very sick patient whilst getting very little support or direction from his colleague. Chris was working with an experienced paramedic (Jim) but had received little encouragement all shift. We have just attended an incident with a sick patient, gosh I felt sorry for Chris, as he couldn't do a thing right. Tempers are now fraught with tension between them both. I was tempted to step in but didn't. Another insider outsider dilemma! |
| Professional Identity | Whilst on route to the second call of the shift, Jim who was driving the ambulance, promptly turns the radio volume on full. We then continued to drive to the call with both the ambulance cab side window fully open whilst music (Meat Loaf's-Bat out-of-Hell) pounded the surrounding area as we sped through the streets. Whilst Alan and Jim accompanied the music by singing as loud as possible. |

*(Continued)*

*Table 4.4* (Continued)

| Colour categorisation of data clusters | Example of my fieldnote and interview dataset |
|---|---|
| Institutionalisation | *Throughout my observational shifts as a researcher, I recognised experienced members of the ambulance service (paramedics) insignia (wearing badges) on their uniforms. These badges were new to me and I needed to understand what they represented. I subsequently discovered, they represented a period of long service, such as 10, 20, & 30 years' service of the individual to the ambulance service. As an 'insider' researcher this was of interest to me.* |
| Professional Identity | *Members of the public appeared to expect and accept some kind of order to be restored, to an often-chaotic scene, as we (ambulance crew) arrived at the emergency call.* |
| Institutionalisation | *It was very evident from the beginning of the shift that (Tina), the paramedic, wasn't comfortable having a student with her, I spoke with (Amy) the student who hadn't worked with Tina before. It was clear that it wasn't going to be an easy shift and I felt sorry for (Amy) as the shift progressed, as she often found herself in challenging and unsupportive situations. I had time to speak with (Amy) at the end of shift and it was of no surprise that she hated the shift, stating: 'How do you (the university) expect us (students) to work like this, you know we had some sick patients this evening and I got no support from her (Tina the paramedic). I feel like just giving the lot up'.* |
| Institutionalisation | *I observed students returning to university and discussing their practice placement experience back in the classroom setting. This was free time for students to share their practice experiences. I was struck by the sense of excitement and their sense of community within their discussions. There was a distinct sense of being 'street wise' and authoritative, as they discussed their role as paramedics, not necessarily as students. There were areas of elitism demonstrated within their discussion, often in connection with their mentor or station complex or at times themselves.* |

from the data by refining and clarifying the interactions of participants (Patton, 2002). To help accommodate and manage the patterns formed from the thematic analyses, we initially identified recurring concepts. The ethnographic data obtained from the face-to-face interviews, observational fieldnotes, and reflections were subsequently managed utilising a blend of both manual and computer techniques. Data from my observational fieldnotes, along with data voice recordings from interviews and my reflections, were supported with electronic software to assist in managing the dataset. The supporting software helps to enhance and enrich data through electronic management of the dataset, as noted by Schonfelder (2011). The supporting software is not there to replace, alter, or compensate for the data analysis, as this takes place manually by the researcher using thematic analysis and identifying themes which may be common through the dataset (Hammersley, 1993). It is only then that the supporting software assists in the management of data, as it helps to sort and manage the data from the various themes already identified and appropriately coded by the researcher (Adler & Adler, 2008) systematically and thematically.

We drew on van Maanen's (1990) narrative tales, to portray and elicit the ethnographer's journey. The data is viewed through the lens of a researcher, rather than a paramedic, although I balanced my interpretation with the participants' explanations of events and my experience as a paramedic. We drew comfort from the literature along with my knowledge and understanding of the clinical workplace. The analysis of my data was such that it was difficult to ascertain what I had initially seen. We were then able to interpret this and offer an illustration and description of enculturation into the ambulance service workplace, as we were eventually able to understand my observations and recording, as I moved beyond the shallow aspect of the research to an in-depth position, allowing me to assimilate any discordancy to the overall meaning within a larger context. By keeping in mind the notion of enculturation, as a central premise of my study, we were able to forge together elements of data to help make sense and unravel meanings of my fieldnotes. We were aware of Savin-Baden's (2004) example that there are multiple meanings in many situations which may differ for both the participant and researcher. We were able to draw together various patterns, trends, experiences, situations, and behaviours, to help weave together and illuminate glimpses of enculturation which revealed something authentic and significant.

To undertake an 'ethnography requires at a minimum, some understanding of the language, concepts, categories, practices, rules, and beliefs, used by members of the group being observed' (van Maanen, 2011: 13). We had jurisdiction over the translation of my data, yet I also had to acknowledge the various interviews and dialogue which took place throughout the research. This, to a degree, authenticated the data, as I interwove various elements of literature with that of my findings. I was able to ensure a resemblance with other earlier forms of studies and ethnographies carried out on paramedics. For example, the work of Metz (1981) and his findings that crews would speculate on the type of patient they were attending whilst on route to the emergency call, and McCann et al.'s (2013) work highlighting how they found one of their researchers being hurried out of the hospital by an ambulance manager, along with the ambulance crew, illustrate some of the frustrations and tensions experienced by crews. Any suspicion of my personal experiences as a paramedic corrupting or altering the integrity of the data was minimalised and, if possible, excluded from various elements of transcribed data. We did this by comparing and checking my fieldnotes with students' interview data wherever possible. The remaining components of data collectively formed a comprehensive illustration of enculturation found within the NHS ambulance service trust where this ethnography was conducted.

### 4.9.6 Conclusions

In conclusion, the ethnography used in this study provides a rich, meaningful insight into an area of student paramedic education, as they move from a position of university studies to become enculturated into the pre-hospital emergency care environment of the paramedic workplace. By undertaking an ethnographic approach, we were able to delve into an area of interest, often unseen and neglected by some studies. The ethnography has provided a method of enquiry which explores both student paramedics and experienced paramedics, along with a framework which provides 'an interpretive and exploratory story about a group of people and their sociality, cultural and behavioural accounts' (Madden, 2017: 16). Concepts which integrate a conceptual framework and support one another express their corresponding phenomena, and, as suggested by Jabareen (2009), create a framework-specific philosophy. The ontological, epistemological, and methodological assumptions are drawn out from the study as knowledge of the way things have become apparent to the researcher (Guba & Lincoln, 1994) illuminating the real-world experience.

We knew what we were trying to achieve and needed a starting point as the premise of the work. The literature provides accounts of paramedics and EMTs being investigated and studied, often in the USA, Canada, and Australia. O'Reilly (2009: 189) argues: 'The ethnographer, considers the politics of representation; to reclaim some authority for the academic ethnographer, whilst retaining what was beneficial, intelligent, and insightful from the reflexive turn'. As researchers, we wanted a stringent research process. We thought about O'Reilly's views and how these may impact on data collection and how she interprets this. We needed to understand from my research the complexities of multiple situations. Brewer (2000: 17) initially alerted us to ethnography, as a descriptive account of 'telling it like it is from the inside'. Becker (1970) reaffirmed the use of ethnography from his seminal works. Significant factors drawn from the literature guided us to adopt observational field studies embedded within ethnographic principles as the predominant methodological approach for the research. Hammersley and Atkinson (2006) reminded us of the importance to approach the subject with a clear understanding of the theoretical underpinning of ethnography.

It was important to reflect, with a degree of accuracy and authenticity, what really goes on in the ambulance service, as students attend their clinical work placements. This approach, as Brewer (2000) calls, is analytical realism. Altheide and Johnson (1998) argue that analytical realism is situated, and that the social world is an interpreted world, rather than a literal one, suggesting constructs are drawn from a world view rather than accepts it for what it is. Therefore, the ethnographer focuses on obtaining various perspectives on the participants' social realities and analytical realisms and acknowledges that most fields have multiple perspectives, voices, and lenses in which to view the activity, reaffirming Altheide and Johnson's (2011) suggestion that the ethnographer reports this and identifies his/her own voice within this.

### 4.9.7 Overview of the chapter

In this chapter, we have identified and critically reviewed the use of ethnographic methods. The advantages and prevalence of studying the lived experiences of participants become evident, as the often taken-for-granted assumptions and understandings are challenged, as the everyday nuances, intricacies, and unseen, unheard, and unknown aspects of the workplace are exposed. We provided and justified details of the research process which included recruitment of participants, along with some of the challenges associated with this process, ethical considerations, data collecting tools, and pilot study, along with the structure and credibility of data analysis.

The chapter concluded with a discussion on ethnography which served to highlight my position as a healthcare professional and academic researcher along with my personal position, which uncovered various beliefs, values, ethical dilemmas, and experiences. These contributed to and influenced the research process which subsequently shaped the interpretation of my observations to contextualise the situated meaning and an in-depth understanding of ethnography.

### References

Abdullah, A. (1992) 'The influence of ethnic values on managerial practices in Malaysia', *Malaysian Management Review*, 27(1), pp. 3–18.

Adler, P. A. & Adler, P. (1987) *Membership Roles in Field Research*, 6th ed. Newbury Park, CA: SAGE Publishing.

Adler, P. A. & Adler, P. (2008) 'Of rhetoric & representation: The four faces of ethnography', *The Sociological Quarterly*, 49(1), pp. 1–30.

Altheide, D. L. & Johnson, J. M. (1998) *Collecting and Interpreting Qualitative Material*. London: SAGE Publishing.

Altheide, D. L. & Johnson, J. M. (2011) *Sage Hand Book of Qualitative Research*, 4th ed. Cited in Denzine, S. & Lincoln, N. K. Los Angeles/London/New Delhi/Singapore/Washington, DC: SAGE Publishing.

Atkinson, P., Coffey, A., Delamont, S., Lofland, J. & Lofland, L. (2007) *Handbook of Ethnography*, 2nd ed. Thousand Oaks, CA/London/New Delhi/Singapore: SAGE Publishing.

Becker, H. (1970) *Sociological Work: Methods and Substance*. London: Routledge, p. 133.

Becker, H., Geer, B., Hughes, C. E. & Strauss, L. A. (1961) *Boys in White*. New Brunswick, NJ/London: Transaction Books.

Brabbie, E. (1989) *The Practice of Social Research*. London: Wadsworth.

Brewer, J. D. (1991) *Inside the RUC.* Oxford: Oxford University Press.

Brewer, J. D. (2000) *Ethnography – Understanding Social Research.* Berkshire/New York: Open University Press.

Burgess, R. G. (1983) *In the Field.* London: Allen & Unwin.

Burgess, R. G. (1985) *Field Methods in the Study of Education.* Edited by R. G. Burgess. London/Philadelphia, PA: Falmer Press Ltd.

Coffey, A. & Atkinson, P. (1996) *Concepts and Coding. Making Sense of Qualitative Data: Complementary Research Strategies.* Thousand Oaks, CA/London/New Delhi/Singapore: SAGE Publishing, pp. 26–53.

Cohen, A. & Golan, R. (2007) 'Predicting absenteeism and turnover intentions by past absenteeism and work attitudes', *Career Development International,* 12(5), pp. 416–432.

Cohen, H. A. (1981) *The Nurse's Quest for a Professional Identity.* Menlo Park: Addison-Wesley Publishing Company, Medical/Nursing Division, University of Michigan.

Corman, K. M. (2016) 'Street medicine – Assessment work strategies of paramedics on the front lines of emergency health services', *Journal of Contemporary Ethnography,* 46(5), pp. 600–623.

Corman, K. M. (2017) *Paramedics on and off the Streets-Emergency Medical Services in the Age of Technological Governance.* Toronto/Buffalo/London: University of Toronto Press.

Craft, A. & Jeffrey, B. (2008) 'Creativity and performativity in teaching and learning: Tensions, dilemmas, constraints, accommodations and synthesis', *British Educational Research Journal,* 34(5), pp. 577–584.

Creswell J. W. (2008) *Research Design-Qualitative, Quantitative, and Mixed Methods Approaches,* 3rd ed. Thousand Oaks, CA/New Delhi/London/Singapore: SAGE Publishing.

Crotty, J. & Crotty, S. (2004) 'Social construction and policy implementation: Inmate health as a public health issue', *Social Science Quarterly,* 85(2), pp. 240–256.

Denzin, N. (2017) *Sociological Methods: A Sourcebook.* London/New York: Routledge.

Denzin, N. & Lincoln, Y. (2002) *The Qualitative Inquiry Reader.* London: SAGE Publishing.

Denzin, N. & Lincoln, Y. (2008) *The Discipline and Practice of Qualitative Research.* London: SAGE Publishing.

Diamond, T. (2008) 'Participant observation in institutional ethnography', *Institutional Ethnography as Practice,* pp. 45–63.

Draper, J. (2015) 'Ethnography: Principles, practice and potential', *Nursing Times,* 29(36), pp. 36–41.

Gagliardi, A. R., Perrier, L., Webster, F., Leslie, K., Bell, M., Levinson, W., Rotstein, O., Tourangeau, A., Morrison, L., Silver, I. L. & Straus, S. E. (2009) 'Exploring mentorship as a strategy to build capacity for knowledge translation research and practice: Protocol for a qualitative study', *Implementation Science,* 4(1), pp. 1–8.

Geertz, C. (1973) *The Interpretation of Cultures.* New York, NY: Basic Books.

Givati, A., Markham, C. & Street, K. (2018) 'The bargaining of professionalism in emergency care practice: NHS paramedics and higher education', *Advances in Health Science Education,* 23, p. 353.

Guba, E. G. (1989) *The Paradigm Dialog.* Alternative Paradigm Conference, March 1989, Indiana University, School of Education, San Francisco, CA, USA, 1990, p. 18.

Guba, E. G. & Lincoln, Y. (1994) 'Competing Demands in Qualitative Research', in N. K. Denzin & Y. S. Lincoln (Eds.), *Handbook of Qualitative Research*. London/Thousand Oaks, CA/New Delhi/Singapore: Sage Publications, Inc., pp. 105–117.

Hammersley, M. (1993) *Social Research – Philosophy, Politics and Practice*. London/Thousand Oaks, CA/New Delhi: SAGE Publications.

Hammersley, M. (2018) 'Ethnomethodological criticism of ethnography', *Qualitative Research*, 19(5), pp. 578–593.

Hammersley, M. & Atkinson, P. (2006) *Ethnography: Principles in Practice*, 3rd ed. London: Routledge, pp. 1–3.

Hawker, S. (2006) *Concise Oxford English Dictionary*, 3rd ed rev. Oxford/New York: Oxford University Press.

Health and Care Professions Council, Standards of Conduct, Performance and Ethics. (2016) https://www.hcpc-uk.org/globalassets/resources/standards/standards-of-conduct-performance-and-ethics.pdf?v=637171211260000000

Higginbottom, G. M. A. (2004) 'Sampling issues in qualitative research', *Nurse Researcher* (through 2013), 12(1), p. 7.

Jabareen, Y. (2009) 'Building a conceptual framework: Philosophy, definitions, and procedure', *International Journal of Qualitative Methods*, 8(4), pp. 49–62.

Kelly, A. A. (1955) *A Theory of Personality: The Psychology of Personal Constructs*. London: Norton.

Kielmann, K. (2012) 'The ethnographic lens', in *Health Policy and Systems Research: A Methodology Reader*. Geneva: Alliance for Health Policy and Systems Research, World Health Organisation, WHO Library Cataloguing-in-Publication Data, pp. 235–252. ISBN 978 92 4 150313 6.

Koch, T. (1996) 'Implementation of a hermeneutic inquiry in nursing: Philosophy, rigour and representation', *Journal of Advanced Nursing*, 24(1), pp. 174–184.

Kuhn, T. S. (1996) *The Structure of Scientific Revolution*, 3rd ed. Chicago: University of Chicago Press.

Kvale, S. (1996) 'The 1,000-page question', *Qualitative Inquiry*, 2(3), pp. 275–284.

Labaree, R. V. (2002) 'The risk of "going observationalist": Negotiating the hidden dilemmas of being an insider participant observer', *Qualitative Research*, 2(1), pp. 97–122.

Lave, J. & Wenger, E. (1991) *Situated Learning: Legitimate Peripheral Participation*. Cambridge/New York/Melbourne/Cape Town/Singapore/Sao Paulo/Delhi: Cambridge University Press.

LeCompte, M. D. & Schensul, J. J. (1999) *Designing and Conducting Ethnographic Research* (Vol. 1). Plymouth: Rowman Altamira.

Lipsky, M. (2010) Street-Level Bureaucracy Dilemmas of the Individual in Public Services. New York: Russel Sage Foundation.

Lynn, C. D., Howells, M. E. & Stein, M. J. (2018) 'Family and the field: Expectations of a field-based research career affect researcher family planning decisions', *PLoS One*, 13(9), p. e0203500.

Madden, R. (2017) *Being Ethnographic: A Guide to the Theory and Practice of Ethnography*, 2nd ed. London/Thousand Oaks, CA/New Delhi/Singapore: SAGE Publishing.

Mann. S. J. (1992) 'Telling a life story: Issues for research', *Management Education and Development*, 23(3), pp. 271–280.

McCann, L., Granter, E., Hyde, P. & Hassard, J. (2013) 'Still blue-collar after all these years? An ethnography of the professionalisation of emergency work', *Journal of Management Studies*, 50(5), pp. 750–774.

Metz, L. D. (1981) *Running Hot-Structure and Stress in Ambulance Work*, 1st ed. Edited by L. D. Metz. Cambridge, MA: Abt Books.

O'Reilly, K. (2009) *Key Concepts in Ethnography*. London/Thousand Oaks, CA/New Delhi/Singapore: SAGE Publishing.

Palmer, E. (1983) ' "Trauma Junkie" and street work: Occupational behaviour of paramedics and emergency medical technicians', *Journal of Contemporary Ethnography, Urban Life*, 12(2), pp. 162–183.

Palmer, E. (1989) 'Paramedic performance', *Sociological Spectrum*, 9, pp. 211–225.

Patton, M. (2002) *Qualitative Research and Evaluation Methods*, 3rd ed. London: SAGE Publishing.

Pike, K. (1967) *Language in Relation to a Unified Theory of the Structure of Human Behaviour*, 2nd ed. The Hague/Paris: Mouton and Co.

Rankin, J. M. & Campbell, M. L. (2006) *Managing to Nurse: Inside Canada's Health Care Reform*. Toronto, ON: University of Toronto Press.

Savin-Baden, S. (2004) 'Achieving reflexivity: Moving researchers from analysis to interpretation in collaborative Inquiry', *Journal of Social Work*, 18(3), pp. 365–378.

Schon, D. (1983) *The Reflective Practitioner. How Professionals Think in Action*. London: Temple Smith.

Schonfelder, W. (2011) 'CAQDAS and qualitative syllogism logic-NVivo 8 and MAX-QDA10 compared', *Forum: Qualitative Social Research*, 12(1).

Schwandt, T. A. (2007) *The Sage Dictionary of Qualitative Inquiry*. Thousand Oaks, CA/London/New Delhi/Singapore: SAGE Publishing.

Searle, J. (1995) *The Construction of Social Reality*. New York, NY: Free Press.

Seifert, T. A., Goodman, K. M., Lindsay, N., Jorgensen, J. D., Wolniak, G. C., Pascarella, E. T. & Blaich, C. (2008) 'The effects of liberal arts experiences on liberal arts outcomes', *Research in Higher Education*, 49(2), pp. 107–125.

Spradley, J. (1979) 'Asking descriptive questions', *The Ethnographic Interview*, 1, pp. 44–61.

van Maanen, J. (1990) 'Great moments in ethnography. An editor's introduction', *Journal of Contemporary Ethnography*, 19(1), pp. 3–7.

van Maanen, J. (2011) *Tales of the Field: On Writing Ethnography*, 2nd ed. Chicago/London: The University of Chicago.

van Maanen, J. (2015) 'The present of things past: Ethnography and career studies', *Human Relations,* 68(1), pp. 35–53.

van Teijlingen, E. & Hundley, V. (2002 *Nursing Standards*. fretboardblueprint.com

Walford, G. (2003) *Introduction: British Private Schools: Research on Policy and Practice*. London: Woburn Pres, pp. 1–8.

Walford, G. (2008) *How to do Educational Ethnography*. London: Tufness Press.

# 5    Findings

## 5.1 Introduction

In this chapter, the findings are categorised into three broad emerging themes. These themes consist of student work experience, paramedic professional identity, and institutionalisation. These themes sit within, and are influenced, by a subculture, along with a hidden curriculum which it gives rise to, Mulder et al. (2019), also see Hafferty and O'Donnell (2014). The themes weave through the work as both discrete and overt forms of data. They provide ways of understanding many of the intricacies and nuances emerging out of the research (Breen, 2007). The transition of paramedic students, from the classroom to the workplace, is illustrated by examining this change from a framework of enculturation as both a concept and through the lived experience of the paramedic students, as also seen in the work of Grusec and Hastings (2007) on socialisation.

The chapter starts with a section which describes the environment which sets the scene of a typical shift for a paramedic. The aspects of data which make up the three themes and contribute to student enculturation are then discussed, each of which is illustrated using the data collected from the fieldnotes, interviews, reflections, and occasional reports. Working practices are described through extracts from fieldnotes and interview transcripts used throughout the chapter. Whilst collecting the data, experienced paramedics and students sometimes resorted to strong language, jargon, and anecdotes. For the sake of authenticity, where possible these have been retained in the transcripts in this chapter. We have used pseudonyms and fictitious details to disguise the NHS ambulance service trust where the study took place, along with those individuals involved in the study and the university where students were studying. The chapter concludes with a summary of findings.

## 5.2 Setting the scene

In the course of collecting data, paramedics commonly worked in traditional ambulances, known as doubled-crewed vehicles. These doubled crewed ambulances consisted of two people who form the ambulance crew. In

DOI: 10.4324/9781032721408-5

addition, some paramedics worked on alternative forms of response units. These consisted of motorcycles, bicycles, and fast response cars. These alternative forms of response are designed to reach the scene of life-threatening incidents quickly, allowing the paramedic to initiate life support and immediate care to the patient whilst waiting for the doubled crewed ambulance (DCA) to arrive. Only traditional doubled crewed ambulances have the capacity to convey patients to hospital. In addition, paramedics have the support of pre-hospital emergency care physicians if required. These physicians are traditionally attached to air ambulances (helicopters) or fast response units and can support the paramedic with additional critical care interventions, such as anaesthetic agents, pre-hospital surgical procedures, and advanced primary care assessment and treatments. However, it should be recognised that recent developments, such as independent prescribing for paramedics (2019) and the new threshold for paramedic registration (2018), now allow some advanced paramedics and specialist paramedics to undertake various advanced techniques and interventions.

Paramedics also work in multiple sites and situations. This work tended to be chaotic, often unpredictable, and at times threatening and dangerous, whilst illustrating a uniqueness of its own, as no two incidents (999 emergency calls) were the same. These characteristics of paramedic practice are illustrated in the work of Metz (1981), Mannon (1992), Corman (2017), McCann et al. (2013), and Palmer (1989). Consequently, the unpredictable nature of paramedic work can be challenging as each incident is different and can range from critical lifesaving interventions to dealing with minor incidents. However, the majority of the day-to-day work of paramedics lies within the ambulance setting, or *truck, bus, or van* as crews refer to it. Corman (2017) illustrates how Canadian paramedics refer to the ambulance as the *rig*. This is important, as students are immediately drawn to using these insider terms as they provide an indication of acceptance into the community of practice (Lave & Wenger, 1991). Subsequently the ambulance becomes the paramedics' office (Corman, 2017) for the shift. This comprises the driver's cab, which forms the front of the vehicle where the crew will spend most of the day together when not conveying patients to hospital.

The rear of the ambulance, known as the saloon, comprises of a treatment centre, consisting of a trolley bed (stretcher) which is detachable from the interior of the ambulance and removed via the use of a tail lift at the rear of the ambulance, allowing the trolley bed to be taken to the patient if necessary. The remainder of the saloon consists of three small seats, one positioned at the head of the trolley bed facing backwards and used by the paramedic to manage the patient's airway, and the other two seats are perpendicular to the trolley bed but can be rotated forward facing. These seats allow the paramedic to carry out general clinical observations on the patient whilst obtaining patient details.

The saloon of the ambulance also consists of numerous cupboards and shelves containing various pieces of ambulance equipment and kitbags used by the crew depending on the situation they are faced with, for example maternity kit, burns kit, splinting devices, defibrillator, airway suction unit, advance life support (ALS) equipment, paediatric kit, infection control kit, various dressings, and intravenous fluids, and also sealed bags containing therapeutic and controlled drugs along with the paramedic's immediate response bag, consisting of life support equipment, some prescription and controlled medications (drugs), and intravenous fluids. There is also an assortment of lifting devices, such as a carry-chair, folding stretcher, and other lifting aids securely stored in the ambulance saloon.

In addition to the ambulance, there are several other factors which influence the paramedic's daily work; these comprise the various geographic locations of the incident, such as the street, the patient's home, workplace, sports facility, police custody suites, offices, prisons, shopping malls, and transport networks. Their work is also influenced by the people involved in the incident and comprises of casualties, relatives, bystanders, prisoners, first aiders, social workers, other emergency service personnel, and so on. The environment also impacts on their work (Burgess, 2010), such as whether it is a rural or urban area, the weather conditions, time of day or night, and, lastly, the length of their shift. This normally lasts 12 hours, although crews often incur late calls, resulting in 13–14-hour shifts. There is little legislation which restricts the paramedic's hours of operational duty and what legislation is available is weak. Therefore, crews are obligated by their contract of employment not to refuse an emergency call during their allocated shift times, regardless of how many hours they have already worked. The location of each incident varies, although the familiar day-to-day setting of the ambulance remains the same. To exemplify this, a typical 12-hour shift is described in the following.

## 5.3  A typical 12-hour shift

On any one day, the student is attached to a large ambulance complex, comprising of two to three smaller ambulance stations, which we are calling satellite stations (satellites). These stations are situated in relatively close proximity to the main ambulance complex, within a few miles or so. The student works closely with his/her colleague or mentor, although this can often change from day to day resulting in the student not necessarily meeting his/her assigned mentor on a shift rotation. Boychuck Duchscher and Cowin (2004) found similarities with student nurses who enter clinical practice and rotate through various departments and mentors.

The commencement of the paramedic shift consists of checking the equipment stored within the ambulance whilst waiting for the first emergency call. However, the first call is often received within the first few minutes of starting the shift allowing minimal, if any, time to carry out these essential checks which also include the road worthiness of the vehicle. If an emergency call is not assigned after a short period of time, normally 10–15 minutes, the crew would most probably be mobilised out on standby. Standbys consist of dispatching an ambulance to a specific geographic location which is determined by the central ambulance control dispatch centre. This procedure is used when an area of high call volume is received in central ambulance control, who themselves have limited, if any, local resources (ambulances) to send to the scene of the incident. An example could be an area consisting of busy transportation hubs, such as railway stations, shopping malls, or sporting venues.

The crew would set off in the ambulance which often comprises a rather cramped, overheated, stuffy, and scruffy ambulance cab, often with an aroma of stale food and perspiration because of the previous crew's 12+ hours of working together in the front of the vehicle (the cab). In stark contrast is the more clinical setting of the rear of the ambulance (the saloon), where I was seated as researcher (on the airway seat) for much of the time whilst travelling to emergency calls. The saloon afforded a more tranquil environment with adjustable lighting and heating/air-conditioning, as opposed to the noisy cab of the ambulance, which constantly echoed the broken voices of distant radio messages between various ambulance crews and ambulance control centre. The relentless sound of the siren and constant electronic alerts (bleeps and buzzers) arising out of the computur's mobile data terminal (MDT) alerting the crew of an incoming emergency call, a cancellation, an update, or urgent information concerning the incident was an ongoing distraction. In addition, there was the commercial radio station, playing popular music, which many crews liked to play (extract from the fieldnotes in the following helps to illustrate this). At the same time, the data-track navigation system periodically bellowed electronic voice recordings, instructing the driver to turn left, turn right, ahead at the roundabout, or that we had arrived at our destination. This incursion of noise impacts upon the student and paramedic who need to construct a plan of action for when arriving at scene. Corman (2017) refers to the activity and noise generated in the (ambulance) cab as they speedily respond to emergency calls. This makes up the environment in which most of the day-to-day activities take place. It is the crew's mobile office, treatment centre, canteen, patient transport facility, and often playground, as crews become playful and restless, for example teasing each other, throwing paper cups and waste lunch wrappers, and so on.

---

Whilst on route to the second call of the shift, Jim who was driving the ambulance, promptly turns the radio volume on full. We then continued to drive to the call with both the ambulance cab side window fully open whilst music (Meat Loaf's-Bat out-of-Hell) pounded the surrounding area as we sped through the streets. Whilst Alan and Jim accompanied the music by singing as loud as possible (18/08/2013).

Taken from my fieldnotes (18/08/2013).

In the aforementioned paragraphs, we have tried to encapsulate the close community which the student, paramedic, and myself as researcher occupied for the duration of our time together whilst collecting data. This provides a sense of the paramedic environment and coincides with the ethnographic studies of Metz (1981), Mannon (1992), Corman (2017), McCann et al. (2013), and Palmer (1989). The next section contextualises the current situation of the UK paramedics.

## 5.4 Context

As discussed in Chapter 2, the transition and development of the paramedic profession, along with the growing shortage of paramedic practitioners, have led to an exceptionally high increase of inexperienced paramedics entering the workplace (AACE, 2016; COP, 2015; Lovegrove, 2013) which has resulted in a diverse workforce, comprising of international, European, and UK paramedics joining the ambulance service from university or, previously, through direct entry into the ambulance service. I was often struck by the diversity of experience, skill mix, and knowledge of many paramedic practitioners which I observed whilst undertaking the field studies. Such a diverse workforce has the potential to offer significant opportunities, both culturally and socially within the development of the growing profession (AACE, 2016; Kline et al., 2017). This brings a variety of skills and prior knowledge, along with differing practical experiences and educational grounding to the practice setting (Public Health England, 2020). Such opportunities consist of inter-professional working between cultural groups, allowing paramedics to share experiences of their country with that of the UK. Furthermore, the social interaction between practitioners and students can be enhanced by the multi-professional workforce. An example of this is illustrated in my observational fieldnotes in the following. The fieldnotes also illustrates the high regard students can have for experienced paramedics.

---

Whilst travelling back to station, I was interested in the conversation between (James) the student and (Bruce) the paramedic. Bruce was talking about his experience in Australia, compared to that in the UK. It seemed that James was inspired by Bruce's experience, as he continually asked more questions of Bruce whilst we drove back to station. I wondered if this is helping to shape the future workforce. Back on station as we finished our shift, I witnessed James speaking with other Australian paramedics as I drove out the station on route home (01/03/2014).

Taken from my fieldnotes (01/03/2014).

---

So far, this chapter has provided contextual details of the working environment of the paramedic. The chapter will now explore data from the findings. In doing so, it will place the findings under the three predominant themes which I have previously identified but reiterate in this chapter.

## 5.5 Work experience

We found little evidence in my data of any international cohort of practitioners which impacted on the established subculture already present within the ambulance service. Many of the international paramedics originated from Australia and were predominantly newly graduated Australian paramedic students (HCPC, 2016). There were similarities between both new recruits and students with that of the traditional workforce. The similarities which O'Meara, Devenish, Willis et al., and Reynolds imply within the Australian transition from a traditional paramedic training paradigm to one of higher education are synonymous with that of the UK model (O'Meara, 2011; Devenish, 2014; Reynolds, 2004). However, there were tensions between both international new recruits and the UK students and the established traditional paramedic workforce.

## 5.6 Tensions

The tensions found in the data are important as they provide insight and interplay with the working practices inherent throughout the subculture of the ambulance service. The traditional in-house training route, which provided training through the Institute of Health Care and Development (IHCD) training award, formed the established entry route for paramedics prior to graduate entry. The demise of the IHCD training award has become a contentious issue amongst many experienced staff (old-timers). Previously, training for the experienced old-timers consisted of a period of 8–12 weeks and lacked much of the scientific and educational models used in today's graduate programmes, as also seen in the work of Donaghy (2010), Devenish (2014), and O'Meara (2011). This disparity of knowledge results in tensions between experienced staff and recruits. I encountered tangible and deeply pragmatic issues whilst collecting data. Students were often unable to defend their position within the practice setting. Experienced staff would not, or did not, recognise or accept graduate paramedics, therefore students were required to comply with traditional norms and practices. These sometimes consisted of deviant, ethical, and moral dilemmas, not conducive to that expected by the professional body, health services, regulator, and the academic community. The introduction of a graduate degree was seen as a catalyst for change, based on the belief that professionalisation would inevitably follow. This is expressed in various reports and academic publications, examples of which are provided in the following.

Extract from the Paramedic Evidence Based Education Project (PEEP):

The role of paramedics has become increasingly important over recent years, with growing expectation for ambulance services to deliver the right care in the right place first time. As early as 2005, it was recognised that investing in the clinical development of the frontline ambulance staff would yield significant benefits for patient outcomes and to the health economy.

(Lovegrove, 2013: 13)

Extract from College of Paramedics:

The transition from a training paradigm into the world of further and higher education has already moved us to the next era of preparing the profession to fulfil its role in a modern health service.

(Furber, 2008: 2)

Regulation should act as a driver to quality improvement, as well as taking action against those who do not meet accepted standards. This is the litmus test – are we as regulators concerned with quality – our own and those regulated by us – or not? Regulatory bodies must be constantly self-critical, reflective, emulating the high standards of professionalism of those they regulate.

(van der Gaag & Donaghy, 2013: 10)

Journal of Paramedic Practice:

Over the past 15 years, the training and education of technicians and paramedics has seen a shift from the more traditional approach initiated by the Institute of Healthcare and Development (IHCD) towards an academic route, developed in association with Higher Education Institutions (HEIs). This shift reflects the curriculum framework put forward by the British Paramedic Association (BPA), now the College of Paramedics (COP), which acts as an educational basis for future paramedic education. The essential transition from training to education is viewed as key for the future of ambulance service delivery.

(Donaghy, 2010: 528)

Early recognition and development of the professional body, along with the transition into higher education, were meant to create a professional group of practitioners, although it is unclear that this had taken place. This abstract concept has not yet been fully understood or embraced within the profession. The aspirations expressed earlier were somewhat disconnected from the realities of practice. I provide examples here taken from the fieldnotes to help illustrate this.

> Tony, the student, gave a number of examples of events where there had been problems. Each event has a student paramedic at the heart of the incident. We spoke about 'dangerous Jim', a paramedic, whom I had rode out with just a few weeks previously with another student whilst collecting data. Tony referred to dangerous Jim as 'fucking Coco the clown'. I asked why Coco the clown? Jim answered, 'he is a fucking menace and difficult to work with. He's just a clown' (12/04/2013).
> Taken from my fieldnotes (12/04/2013).

> I am on a Saturday nightshift with Liz (student). Liz is not sure who her colleague (crew mate) will be tonight. In the meantime, Liz and I go to check the vehicle (ambulance) which has been allocated to us for the shift. Halfway through the checks, two experienced paramedics (old timers) approach us and demand that they use this vehicle tonight (the vehicle was new). In the absence of Liz's crewmate, I tried to explain that this vehicle had been allocated to us and we are halfway through the checks. This had no impression on the two 'old timers' experienced paramedics, so Liz and I changed vehicles! (05/09/2014).
> Taken from my fieldnotes (05/09/2014).

The next two examples in the following help illustrate the subtle pedagogy emerging from the data. The salience of the subtle aspects of subculture drew the students into traditional working processes and practices, which were not taught in the formal university classroom. The first student was unable to address the situation in which he found himself and accepted the perverse and hostile situation for the duration of the 12-hour shift. The second example provides a paradox. Here the student was allowed to treat a very sick patient whilst the experienced paramedic (old-timer) showed little, if any, interest in either the patient's clinical condition or the student paramedic's inability and lack of experience to manage the complex clinical presentation.

> As soon as I started the shift it was apparent that there were tensions between the crew. When I had the opportunity, I spoke with the student (Tom), I asked him why such hostility between them both (him and his

crewmate) the paramedic (Bill). Tom threw his eyes to the back of his head and said, 'John (researcher), he is a knob, Bill doesn't want to be here, and he takes it out on us (students) although he is okay with his old stooges' (I took this to mean the experienced old hands) 'and he seems okay with you John (researcher), but that's because you are a visitor' (13/04/2013).

Taken from my fieldnotes (13/04/2013).

I could see the student (Chris) struggling to cope with the enormity of dealing with a very sick patient whilst getting very little support or direction from his colleague. Chris was working with an experienced paramedic (Jim) but had received little encouragement all shift. We have just attended an incident with a sick patient, gosh I felt sorry for Chris, as he couldn't do a thing right. Tempers are now fraught with tension between them both. I was tempted to step in but didn't. Another insider outsider dilemma!

Taken from my fieldnotes (17/05/2013).

This unprofessional and often disparate behaviour remained evident. There was hostility towards students who did not conform. By not challenging some of the taken-for-granted behaviours displayed by the experienced staff, students were provided with a degree of acceptance into the community of practice, which Lave and Wenger (1991) note. Notwithstanding this, non-conformity resulted in students being ostracised from the ambulance station banter and subsequent community. Another extract from the fieldnotes here provides examples of this.

On route to hospital, I asked the student (Mark) if he had experienced any resentment when he started as a student, some three years ago. His response was: 'Man, you can't believe it, I was ridiculed and abused when I started and I had to learn to live with it, you can't change the "die-hards" you really can't'. I asked him if he could give any specific examples. He referred to an incident in the crew room (watch-room) where he was challenged by two 'old hands' not to make trouble or else! I asked Mark what he thought they meant by this, he said, 'They would have taken me round the back of station and knocked the living shit out of me probably' (18/05/2013).

Taken from my fieldnotes (18/05/2013).

I experienced some hostility and an uneasy atmosphere when I arrived at an ambulance station for my observational shift. The following extract gives an illustration of this.

> As I entered the watch room, my reception appeared somewhat frosty, old-timers not really encouraging me to 'feel welcome' or allow for any introductions, there was tension and I felt very much an outsider within an organisation which I had worked in for the past 30+ years (12/04/2013).
> Taken from my fieldnotes (12/04/2013).

I also found tension between stations, and between paramedics on fast response vehicles (first responders), an example of which is illustrated here, taken from the fieldnotes.

> The next call involved a first responder arriving on scene prior to our arrival; the responder appeared a little agitated, had little to say to us and was quite rude to the crew. I wondered why this might have been, clearly, we were all trying our best for the patient! Why such hostility? I offered to assist the first responder with carrying his equipment back to the response car, but he refused. There appeared to be no apparent reason for this negative response to the crew or myself (12/04/2013).
> Taken from my fieldnotes (12/04/2013).

Tensions between students and paramedics became somewhat normalised. By normalised we draw on Armitage (2010) to help illustrate this as a means in which students became accepting of the behaviour and culture of the workplace. I found students were exposed to numerous and various degrees of interaction with colleagues, mentors, managers, and other healthcare professionals when attending practice placements, some of which resulted in negative experiences, as illustrated in the observations here.

> It was very evident from the beginning of the shift that (Tina), the paramedic, wasn't comfortable having a student with her. I spoke with (Amy) the student who hadn't worked with Tina before. It was clear that it wasn't going to be an easy shift and I felt sorry for (Amy) as the

shift progressed, as she often found herself in challenging and unsupportive situations. I had time to speak with (Amy) at the end of shift and it was of no surprise that she hated the shift, stating:

> 'How do you (the university) expect us (students) to work like this, you know we had some sick patients this evening and I got no support from her (Tina the paramedic). I feel like just giving the lot up' (08/06/2014).

Taken from my fieldnotes (08/06/2014).

There were limited number of mentors, given the number of students attending clinical practice placements and requiring mentorship. Mentors who were available were not always keen to accommodate students for the shift. I found this situation difficult to understand. The partnership agreement between the NHS ambulance service and university requires the ambulance trusts to provide both a positive and a meaningful student experience. Therefore, the agreement stipulates the standards required by both parties to ensure students received a positive educational practice experience (HCPC, 2019). This is an example of where policy and bureaucracy do not reflect the reality of the practice setting, like that which Lipsky (2010) found in his work on housing officers and police officers. I found there were tensions and resentment within the organisation which spanned all aspects of the student experience and working environment. The next section of this chapter highlights the more serious forms of tension that were uncovered throughout the data.

## 5.7 Harassment, inequality, and bullying

We found a hidden curriculum exists which produces a pedagogy far removed from that of university education and professional expectations. The type of behaviour associated with harassment and equality depicted within the research was often covert and had similarities with other uniformed, authoritarian services seen in the work of Coyne et al. (2004), Boychuck Duchschernd and Cowin (2004), and Cowin and Hengstberger-Sims (2004). I found claims of bullying and harassment of staff and students by peers, middle managers, and senior managers. Boychuck Duchscher and Cowin (2004) found that senior nursing staff displayed contempt for newly qualified staff at best and bullying at worse.

A subsequent visit by the Care Quality Commission (CQC, 2015: 39) into the NHS ambulance service trust, where the study was conducted, reported '[s]ignificant concerns about a reported culture of bullying and harassment in parts of the organisation'. There were episodes where harassment and bullying were evident throughout several transcripts which provide some context in which bullying took place (Zapf & Einarsen, 2003). There was also evidence of racism. I provide an example here to help illustrate this (Nabib et al., 2019).

Whilst the student (Janet) and her crew mate, (Asher) were in the watch-room with colleagues, an experienced (old-timer, Tom) paramedic asked who would like a cup of tea. Several colleagues within the watch room replied and said they would like a cup of tea. The experienced paramedic then specifically asked if Asher would also like tea. Asher refused tea, stating 'he was observing Ramadan and that he would not be taking any food or drinks (other than water) whilst at work today'. I observed how the experienced paramedic then focused in on Asher's response. The experienced paramedic continued to mock Asher's views and beliefs and jested to his colleagues, to get Asher a huge cake as 'Asher was observing fucking Ramadan, so get him a big fuck off cake'. Although this rant appeared to be taken in good humour and in a jovial manner by Asher, and other members of staff, as they all appeared to accept the so-called banter. After dealing with the first patient and whilst on route to hospital, I was able to talk to Asher about the previous events which had occurred on the station. I asked Asher how he felt about the so-called banter within the watch-room, and especially about Ramadan. Asher gave a little laugh and said that he must accept it, 'I wear a green uniform like other colleagues' he said, 'it doesn't really matter, although Ramadan is clearly very important to me, I just have to accept this kind of banter, there is no other way'. Asher again gave a little nervous laugh and continued to drive to hospital

Taken from my fieldnotes (12/04/2013).

I provide an example in the following which illustrates unprofessional behaviour bordering on sexism and depicts the hidden subculture inherent throughout the study. Tangherlini (2000: 46) describes these behaviours in his study as 'interacting with a cast of characters so utterly diverse that no Hollywood scriptwriter could ever do justice to'.

Whilst in the watch-room (crew room) beginning our shift, there was a mixture of males and females present. One female asked her colleague if she had watched a particular TV programme the previous night and the conversation soon turned to the subject of sex. One particular male, who was rostered onto the adjacent ambulance to ours, stated that, 'he hadn't watched that particular programme on the television the previous night, unlike his colleagues, as he was too busy fucking xxxxxxx' (masturbating). He then went on to talk about how far he could xxx (ejaculate). My student, (Sarah) was in the watch-room and appeared to give a nervous laugh whilst others laughed at the young man's gesture. I found it uncomfortable and disconcerting, listening to this young man talking about this and wondered how other colleagues may have thought. This was interesting and bizarre at the same time, as various crews in the watch-room had no idea who I was, I was not in ambulance service uniform that day, although I had an ambulance identification (ID) card worn around my neck, that would have been difficult to read unless in very close proximity to me. It struck me that I could have been anybody from the ambulance service, yet no regard was given to whom I may be. On the contrary, it appeared that at least three members of the watch-room banter drew on the assumption that they could impress me with their bizarre and outrageous conversations (13/05/2014).

Taken from my fieldnotes (13/05/2014).

I believe, what was happening here, was that the established relationship forged between the experienced paramedic and other crew members was somewhat threatened by my presence in the crew-room, which Devenish (2014) also relates to. A form of authority was being tested, something McLaughlin et al. (2012) illustrate in their work, as do Martimianakis et al. (2009). There was a perceived threat that the paramedic's status and authority was being challenged by my presence, which illustrates how his behaviour and professional identity became an inherent aspect of the data.

We summarise the working practices which students found themselves involved in – racism, sexism, forms of bullying, hostility, and tension between ambulance control and management. The next section continues under the sub-heading of paramedic professional identity.

## 5.8 Paramedic professional identity

The nature of paramedic work often means both student paramedics and paramedics arrive at the incident in a backdrop of hope and relief from those who require their assistance (patients and bystanders). The high visibility of the ambulance, the flashing blue lights and sirens, alerts people of the paramedics' impending arrival. The distinctive green uniform of the paramedic (Lovegrove and Davis 2013) and other ambulance personnel, such as emergency medical technicians (EMTs) and emergency care assistants (ECAs), along with the calm, calculated way paramedics operated whilst collecting the data, gave them a distinctive identity, which Lovegrove and Davis (2013) believe are symbolic in their workplace. This symbol or status appeared to manifest itself as a form of perceived authority and power whilst dealing with emergency calls (Devenish et al., 2016). Although theorising these concepts in this thesis would be challenging, as it is argued by McNamee and Glasser (1987: 79) that '[n]umerous definitions and conceptualisations of power have been identified', perhaps the most effective means of understanding the power concept of the paramedic for this thesis is from Corman's (2017) study on Canadian paramedics, who also found that the public appeared to want and expect the paramedics to take charge, control, and supervise the situation once they arrive on scene. I found that some experienced paramedics and students metaphorically drew on characters within film and media to express their perceived position within the social structure of the paramedic role, as the following extract helps to illustrate.

---

I am with Harry the student and Dave the paramedic for this shift. I had no sooner started the shift with them when we received a call to a road traffic collision (RTC), a person knocked down. Both Harry & Dave appeared excited and glad to get a 'good' job. As we started our journey with the blue lights and sirens on, Harry promptly stuck his arm and hand out straight towards the top of the ambulance windscreen and shouted, 'don't worry, superman is on his way', whilst Dave the paramedic corrected his student (Harry) by informing him that it was more like Batman and Robin (14/05/2014).

Taken from my fieldnotes (14/05/2014).

---

Their obsession of the role typically reflected their behaviour in station and whilst in the ambulance, as Tangherlini (2000) also notes in his study, as paramedics and students compared themselves to larger-than-life superheroes.

## 5.9 Authority and power

A form of power relations was inherent within the bureaucratic, quasi-military style organisation of the ambulance service which McCann et al. (2013), Corman (2017), and Wankhade (2015) also experienced, as they studied the organisational culture of the ambulance service. This was replicated throughout my data. One example depicts how long-serving paramedics proudly displayed their long service emblems (badges), whilst other elements of their uniform remained unkempt and scruffy.

---

Throughout my observational shifts as a researcher, I recognised experienced members of the ambulance service (paramedics) insignia (wearing badges) on their uniforms. These badges were new to me, and I needed to understand what they represented. I subsequently discovered, they represented a period of long service, such as 10-, 20-, & 30-years' service of the individual to the ambulance service. As an 'insider' researcher this was of interest to me (05/11/2013).

Taken from my fieldnotes (05/11/2013).

---

> When asking one old-timer why he wore this insignia, his reply was:
> 'Well, you get nothing from this setup, so at least I have a badge for my 20 years' service' (05/11/2013 Steve).
> Taken from my fieldnotes (05/11/2013).

The insignia represented the length of service of the practitioners and therefore highlighted their established position within the community. This form of status initiated a degree of authority to students. This was a defining characteristic of many old-timers who curtailed established policies and procedures for traditional ways of working. Lave and Wenger (1991) refer to the work of Becker (1970) as recognising the disastrous consequences and structural constraints which work practices may have for participants. Lipsky (2010) found students were caught between local practices and traditional norms and bureaucratic infrastructure (Grusec & Hastings, 2015). The subculture exposes the vulnerability of students and newcomers into these communities of practice. This appears throughout the data and shows how the hidden curriculum manifests and draws university-educated paramedic degree students into the traditional working ways and established practices inherent within the practice environment.

### 5.9.1 Examples of perceived elitism

We found evidence within the hidden curriculum of what appeared to be a form of professional elitism. I use the term professional elitism in the context of the ambulance and paramedic environment (Lovegrove & Davies, 2013). This was important data which emerged from my findings which needs to be understood. The elitism spanned all sectors of the profession and was evident in several areas of practice, such as certain ambulance stations where specialist teams of paramedics are situated, and where air ambulance providers operate. For example, the following extract taken from the observational fieldnotes displays this behaviour.

> This is the second of three consecutive shifts, in which I am riding out with crews. I am feeling rather weary after working at the university, prior to undertaking the shift. This particular night I am riding out with a comparatively new crew, clearly the student is new and her colleague for the shift has recently finished university and qualified as a newly qualified paramedic (NQP). It is interesting though to see and hear from the onset of the shift, how they appear to have become conditioned into the service jargon and subculture. I was surprised by the response I received

when I ask about the Hazardous Area Response Teams (HART). This is a comparatively new concept for the UK ambulance service whereby specialist crews with specialist equipment and vehicles, respond to incidents involving hazardous environments, such as working at height, confined spaces and hazardous materials. Whilst talking about the HART teams I am met with negativity and verbal innuendos, such as 'they are all lazy sods (Amber), they do nothing and it's a waste of time . . . (Paul)'. This was from both the student and paramedic (11/10/2013).

Taken from my fieldnotes (11/10/2013).

Whilst on my ride-out this particular night with (Sharon) the paramedic and (Julie) the student, we attended quite a serious road traffic collision (RTC). Both Sharon and Julie were excited by the call as we sped off using both our visual and audible warning lights and sirens (commonly known as, blues and two's). I could understand the excitement, this was different from the mundane calls, such as falls, collapses and abdominal (abdo) pains, which we had been dealing with most of the night. As we arrived on scene, we could see both HART and HEMS (in a response car) along with the Fire Service were already on scene. The frustration from Sharon and Julie was very evident, both verbally and behaviourally. After the incident they both expressed their 'negative' views about these specialist teams (09/05/2014). HEMS is the Helicopter Emergency Medical Service.

Observational fieldnotes (09-05-2014)

The dissatisfaction here is because they were denied the interesting cases owing to the presence of the Helicopter Emergency Medical Service (HEMS) which takes supremacy in these types of serious incidents. Extract from interview with paramedic Ben: 'I have no idea what the fuck these teams do (referring to the Hazardous Area Response Team (HARTs), they hardly go out and when they do, they want to take over the poxy job, there're just a waste of fucking time if you ask me' (18–09–14). Extract from student Joe: 'Well I haven't really had any dealings with the Hazardous Area Response Teams (HART) as such, but I can't really see the point of them, you know, what they do, I never see them. No one really likes them John' (researcher) (21/09/2014).

Taken from my fieldnotes (21/09/2014).

The tension expressed here was based on a lack of respect for roles or differing cultures in the ambulance and fire services. There was a distinct sense of resentment, frustration, rejection, and perceived elitism. Paramedics and students would often depict specialist teams as elitists, or a demonstration of elitist behaviours when working together. To try and understand this perception, this section is reflective in nature, as I draw on my own experience to shed light on certain aspects of interpersonal and interagency working. The anatomy of an accident or emergency, by definition, is an unplanned and unknown event, as seen in the work of Metz (1981). Many of these events, or incidents, either require a multiple response, such as additional ambulances, fast response vehicles, or specialist teams, or require a multi-agency response, such as the attendance of the fire service, the police service, and the ambulance service. In addition, other services may also be required, for example lifeboats, coastguard, local authority, and the utility companies such as those responsible for electricity, water, and gas. Tangherlini (2000) also found similar tensions existed between paramedics and fire fighters, or the plugs as paramedics derisively referred to them, in his study. The accumulation of the emergency and essential services arriving at an incident at different times adds to the confusion and often chaotic situation, as everyone goes about their distinct specialist roles. This can sometimes cause tension within individual services and across services, as individuals are not necessarily aware of each other's roles and responsibilities. This can lead to individuals perceiving other roles as elitist and an unwelcoming distraction from their own unique role and responsibility. I draw on Mowforth (1999) to help illustrate this as she implies elitism existed in nursing, as various disciplines perceive each other as elitist, for example intensive care nurses, as opposed to accident and emergency (A&E) nurses, or care of the elderly nursing staff and general nursing. We reviewed the work of Weber (1968) to try and unpack this perception, as he believed alliances were formed within groups, on the understanding of social position and authority. Weber argued that groups have the exclusionary tools in the admission criteria to a particular group. We wondered if this is what was happening here, as many of the ambulance service's 'specialisms', such as the Hazardous Area Response Team (HART), the Helicopter Emergency Medical Service (HEMS), Advanced Paramedics (AP), Primary Care Paramedics (PCP), and Critical Care Paramedics (CCP), require certain unique entry criteria into the group. This results in the group becoming illusive, out of the reach of some paramedics and generally regarded with a degree of contempt and sometimes elitism. Weber describes these restrictions as a process which is often seen in certain developing professions by raising the educational qualifications for applicants. Therefore, the introduction of degree-level education for paramedics, in some respect, may present barriers for some of the experienced (old-timer's) individual's development.

Lisa the paramedic and Julie the student was excited to receive a fire call 'persons reported'. The term 'Persons reported' relates to fire calls whereby the fire has been reported to have potential people inside the building or that people have already been identified as injured from the fire. We made great haste and arrived on scene to see two adult male patients receiving oxygen from the fire and rescue service. Both Lisa and Julie jumped out of the cab of the ambulance and approached the fire fighter and patients. As I was climbing out from the rear of the ambulance, I could see and hear some disagreement taking place with the fire fighter and crew (Lisa & Julie). There was disagreement about the volume of oxygen the patient should be receiving. I watched from a distance and could see and hear how the fire service were claiming seniority over this clinical procedure which was causing such tension for Lisa & Julia (15/02/2014).

Taken from my fieldnotes (15/02/2014).

The following extract provides a further example.

I observed students returning to university and discussing their practice placement experience back in the classroom setting. This was free time for students to share their practice experiences. I was struck by the sense of excitement and their sense of community within their discussions. There was a distinct sense of being 'street wise' and 'authoritative', as they discussed their role as paramedics, not necessarily as students. There were areas of elitism demonstrated within their discussion, often in connection with their mentor or station complex or at times themselves (22/09/2014).

Taken from my fieldnotes (22/09/2014)

Students were keen to assume the identity of paramedics, rather than students. I observed Billy, the student mentioned in the following observational fieldnote, exercise a degree of power and authority at an incident. Lave and Wenger (1991) depict this as full legitimate participation, although this particular paramedic student was still quite new.

The student (Billy) is a very capable and confident student (one may argue verging on cocky and arrogant) Billy, wants to get his point across. He isn't that enthralled with the university, so I stayed clear of mentioning this. We received a call to a Road Traffic Collision (RTC) which appeared to excite Billy; the paramedic (Jimmy) appeared calm and continued to drive to the scene. Upon arrival there were three casualties, although two of them had received very minor injuries. Whilst the other one had sustained whiplash and bruising to the chest, sustained from the seat belt/airbag deployment (a common occurrence following a collision). I witnessed Billy dealing with the minor injured patients and bystanders, his whole demeanour and body language appeared to be one of authority and control. Directing people, assuming control of the incident, stating his intentions to the police officer and so on (12/12/2013).

Taken from my fieldnotes (12/12/2013).

Students related to the traditional practices and norms of day-to-day front-line emergency work which Mannon (1992) and Metz (1981) identify with. The hidden curriculum equipped students with the necessary understanding and confidence to operate in practice, such as that seen in the work of Corman (2017). The traditional working practices and behaviours of experienced paramedics were mirrored in many aspects, as students became increasingly confident and authoritative in many areas of their practice. We provide further examples in the following.

Although communication with the patient was positive, the student (Brian) was very assertive and, at times, his mentor (Charles) was unable to interject into either the communication or patient treatment (12/04/2013).

Taken from my fieldnotes (12/04/2013).

It is interesting watching and listening to these three students at Global City NHS Ambulance Station. I am surprised at the rivalry between them, as they talk about and illustrate the types of calls, they have attended and how they highlight their paramedic colleagues as the 'best', or the 'worst'. They appear to measure both the call they attended on the severity or unusual nature of the incident, which they rate highly. There is competition between their mentors as the students speak of their own mentors' experience and the traumatic discourse of the incident. The language used is often colourful! (10/03/2013).

Taken from my fieldnotes (10/03/2013).

*5.9.2 Deviant behaviour*

We use this sub-heading to help depict some of the unorthodox practices which I witnessed whilst collecting the fieldnotes. There was a clear disparity between the formal classroom learning situated in university and practice learning, which has been suggested by Williams (2005). To understand this knowledge and the influence this had on the students' pedagogy, we found students were drawn into an oppressive, cognitively restrictive working environment. To provide an indication of this dissonance in the experience highlighted in the fieldnotes, we provide two examples of the discourse. One illustrates the damage, resulting from vandalism which was apparent in the vehicles (ambulances) which I rode out on. The other example given in the following is a narrative taken from an official ambulance bulletin which provides an example of unprofessional and offensive behaviours by some staff.

'There have been several occasions recently where the trust (ambulance service) has been brought into disrepute due to drawings of penises as well as scrawling of words, some of which have been interpreted as homophobic slurs on documents around Cowley Cross ambulance station. One occasion, someone had drawn a picture of a penis on an ECG strip and put it back in the Defibrillator/monitor. When an ECG was printed it had a large penis along the patient's heart rhythm. This now forms part of the legal record of the patient's care and was picked up by the consultant in the Accident & Emergency (A&E) department at Cowley Cross hospital. In addition, we have had several internal and external visitors who have commented on the amount of penis drawings, as well as other graffiti, including words intending to cause offence (particularly the word "bender" which was taken to be a homophobic slur) on documents around the mess-room and in particular the male locker room. Again, this now forms part of those visitors' view of the (ambulance service) trust and in particular staff at Cowley Cross station that we allow it to happen. Today, all penis drawings located were covered up or removed, as were any other visual representations which could cause offence. This matter will be the subject of ongoing investigations until the culprit(s) is/are found. Colleagues are reminded that whilst they may wish to add decoration to their locker, the locker remains the property of the trust and any decoration should be non-permanent and should not cause offence. Colleagues are also reminded that all employees have a right to work in an environment free of discrimination or harassment, in particular that which refers to gender or sexuality. Anyone who wishes to provide any information regarding this please get in touch with one of the management team in confidence'.

Extract taken from internal ambulance circular.

*An electrocardiogram's (ECG) rhythm is printed onto graphed paper which prints an electric representation of the patients' heart rhythm. By examining the rhythm against the values of the graph paper, paramedics can diagnose various heart deformities and heart attacks.*

On many of my observational placements I noticed several exposed electrical wires hanging down in the ambulance cab, situated just by the driver's sun visor. My initial enquiry into these exposed wires found hanging in the ambulance cab was one of joyous laughter from crews, followed by an explanation which is illustrated here.

'[W]e (the crews) cut the wires, Len the paramedic tells me. Management had installed small microphones in the cabs of the ambulance, a so-called safety feature management claimed! However, we (crews) cut the wires leaving them hanging. It is a common sight' Len tells me; 'you won't find a vehicle with any of these working he says. They are just spies in the cab', I am told! (12/05/2014).

Len was correct, I never did see any of the actual microphones, just exposed 'bare' wires as highlighted earlier.

Taken from my fieldnotes (12/05/2014).

This form of deviance, bordering on criminal activity, as Shprakh et al. (2019) suggest, typically highlights how both paramedics and students work in a backdrop of accepted subcultural expectations of non-conformity. These norms laid out the recognised behaviour expected within the workplace and community of practice, which Lave and Wenger (1991) imply are forms of acceptance within groups or communities. Becker's (1963) studies on the sociology of deviance conclude that these types of behaviour form a collective action, which he illustrates in his later work as being replicated both within and across the social group or community (Becker, 1964). This suggests that a failure to conform to these deviant behaviours places one outside of the social group, expelled from that community. This is also illustrated by Burt's (1925) and Bell's (2010) early work. This is different from the formal rules and procedures which the ambulance managers expect, and crews find tiresome to follow, especially against a backdrop of a busy working environment, which Lipsky (2010) found in his work. Sharar (2016) suggests people must be drawn into using these formal rules, policed by social agents within society. Here we clarify what we mean by formal rules, as these are not to be confused with that of the accepted norms and behaviours found throughout my data collection. We refer to formal rules as those imposed on crews by either legislation or internal ambulance service policies and procedures, such as patient conveyance policy and procedure or uniform policy. This is different from the day-to-day working practices and norms of behaviours so ingrained in the workplace and evident throughout the data. These taken-for-granted assumptions and behaviours spanned many aspects of the subculture of the ambulance service. The observation from the fieldnotes given here helps to illustrate this.

---

Tim the paramedic was very vocal about the volume of formal documentation that must be completed each and every day. 'The job has become more of an administration role than a caring role', he tells me. 'You near enough need a form to have a shit these days', he tells me! (22/10/2014).
  Taken from my fieldnotes (22/10/2014).

---

In this section of the chapter, we have illustrated some of the behaviours and practices often not seen through media representation of the ambulance service and paramedic profession, yet they were practices and behaviours which were very prominent and widespread throughout the data in the field. The next section of this chapter highlights other areas where traditional working practices were an essential part of working which influenced both experienced staff and students alike.

### 5.9.3 Meal break avoidance and finishing shifts on time

Another feature of a subcultural form of practice which fostered accepted norms of behaviour was the prevalence of meal break avoidance amongst both experienced paramedics and students. We provide an example to help illustrate this practice. Crews would often go out their way to avoid being sent back to their designated ambulance station and stood down for a meal break. The rationale for this behaviour lays in the receipt of a reward for not taking a break. Here crews that were not allocated a meal break would receive a monetary reward of ten pounds in addition to finishing their rostered shift 30 minutes earlier than their planned finishing time. I observed crews driving away from hospitals in the opposite direction to their ambulance station, so they became too far away to be sent back to the station for a meal break. The following example from the fieldnotes provides examples of this widespread practice.

It is 23–00 hours and we are completing the paperwork at Treetop University Hospital. The discussion soon leads to meal breaks and meal break time. The latest opportunity for our break is 00–15 hours, and already plans start to be developed and implemented between the paramedic (Charlotte) & student (Terry) regarding avoidance of the meal break, commonly known within the service as 'meal break avoidance'. According to Charlotte it is vital we (Charlotte) & (Terry) avoid the break so as to finish the shift 30 minutes early (05:30 hours), in addition to receiving £10 for each meal break that is not taken on each shift. Terry & Charlotte seem to think that whilst they are in the Northwest geographical area of the city, they would not receive a meal break. This appears to please them and results in a perceived victory (12/08/2013).

Taken from my fieldnotes (12/08/2013).

After the next call, we were at the hospital waiting to become available, whereby (Ricky), the paramedic activated the mobile data terminal (MDT) to acknowledge that we were now available for another call. Ambulance control acknowledged us and requested that we return to station for a meal break. Ricky appeared annoyed at this suggestion and said to the student (Tracy), 'there is no way we are fucking going back and get a break this time of night'. Ricky then proceeded to drive in the opposite direction from the hospital, which was some distance away from the ambulance station. Tracy gave a nervous laugh and asked if this was okay to do, Ricky was adamant that everyone does this to avoid breaks so I don't see why we shouldn't, he then continued to proceed in the opposite direction to where the ambulance station was situated. There was no challenge or questions from ambulance control and I wondered why they (control) hadn't challenged and questioned us, as they were able to follow the movement of the vehicle via the data tracking device installed within the vehicle. I asked the crew what about control, would they not notice us going in the opposite direction? Ricky suggested that they (ambulance control) are always too busy to notice (18/08/2013).

Taken from my fieldnotes (18/08/2013).

As crews neared the end of their rostered shift a parallel situation to meal break avoidance occurred. Here, I found crews were very keen to finish their shift on time and not receive a late call, often referred to as the *off job* (the last call within the scheduled shift time). Crews would plan, organise, facilitate, and conspire to finish their rostered shift on time. This process begins quite early, normally within 2–3 hours of the end of a crew's shift. Subsequently crews try to work out busy areas known as hot spots to help inform and influence their decisions, such as which hospital to take a patient to, or create a mechanical issue relating to the vehicle or claim that their uniform is damaged or soiled. Consequently, crews tended to want to be in proximity of their ambulance station if possible as they neared the end of their shift, rather than being in some considerable distance from the station. This allowed crews the opportunity to receive the last call of their shift (off job) which they hoped would be in their local area and therefore allowing them to finish their shift on, or near, their scheduled finishing time. Crews vigorously tried to plan their geographic location in the latter stages of their shift, as 999 emergency calls are categorised, depending on the significance of the clinical situation, as described by the person making the 999 call. These calls are then subsequently triaged (arranged in order of clinical priority) in central ambulance control with the aid of computer software programs to help denote the category of call, such as the category known as a red-1 for cardiac arrest and life-threatening emergencies through to green-2 suggesting the patient has no immediate medical life-threatening problems and therefore can receive a delayed response. I found crews would refer to the practice of *off job* with anecdotes. These anecdotes would suggest that the most urgent call you will ever receive is the '*off job*' (last call of the shift), implying that the call would be dealt with quickly to finish the shift, thus suggesting this would be the fastest the ambulance would be driven all shift. The following observations go some way to highlight this.

I was part of a conversation between Mike the paramedic and Tim the student, referring to urgent calls which they had attended. Mike was referring to calls he had received when nearing his finishing time, suggesting there is no more an urgent call than that one. Here 'the ambulance goes faster back to station from the hospital than it ever did going to the emergency call on blue lights and sirens', proclaimed Mike. Both Tim and I laugh at this image (23/06/2014).

Taken from my fieldnotes (23/06/2014).

We spent time 'sitting it out' (waiting at the hospital) whilst we try to gauge our last call (off job). The crew believe they have it sorted and activate the Mobile Data Terminal (MDT) which acknowledges the crew's

availability to ambulance control. As the crew activate the MDT a call is received which is some distance away from our current position, this will not assist the crew to finish on time, they are both questioning the call with ambulance control, calling them on the radio. They must continue with the call for the moment, as no other nearer ambulance is available at this time. Eventually, and to the delight of the crew, the call is cancelled, concurrently an additional call is received immediately, although this is to a closer location which the crew are very pleased with (27/06/2014).
    Taken from my fieldnotes (27/06/2014).

I found experienced paramedics and students had become habituated to this way of working; it appeared to be a kind of survival mechanism, designed to allow crews to finish their shift on time, or with as little dissatisfaction as possible. I found deviant and at times fraudulent practices were taking place to escape the grasp of ambulance control and a possible late call. The following observations help to illustrate some of the practices I witnessed whilst collecting data in the field along with the degree of knowledge required when implementing such strategies.

(Jim) the student turned to speak to me, as (Bill), the paramedic and driver for the day, activated the radio in preparation to speak with control. 'Okay John (researcher), what we do now is think about getting off on time, you must know about this John, we don't want a late job' Jim tells me. Once ambulance control had acknowledged us, Bill told them of a bogus vehicle defect which he claimed had suddenly developed. On our way back to station, in the knowledge that we would not receive another call. Both Jim and Bill spoke about the procedure. It was clear that this is a detailed strategy that crews are aware off. 'Which particular vehicle fault will get us sent back to station is important', Bill said. 'If you get it wrong John, it might mean the vehicle is un-roadworthy (illegal) such as a brake problem for example. Then you are stuck, as they (ambulance control) won't allow you to move the vehicle and that's a right pain in the arse, as you must then wait for a low loader (breakdown recovery vehicle) to arrive and move it back to station for you. This can get you off shift later than the late call itself' (18/06/2013).
    Taken from my fieldnotes (18/06/2013).

Whilst we were driving back to station, Bill (the experienced paramedic) continued to talk about strategies that were used previously, although not so much now due to 'too many poxy close circuit television (CCTV) cameras everywhere', Bill informs me. Bill continued to explain how he would pretend they (the crew) had come across someone in the street (a collapse) and call it into control via the radio. Bill continued to explain, that ambulance control would have to cancel the original call you were going on. I couldn't quite workout where Bill was going with this, I asked him to expand, how would this help? He then explained that 'once they (the crew) had passed their finishing time he would call control and explain that this (phantom) patient had refused treatment and "walked off". They (ambulance control) can't give you another call once you have past your scheduled finishing time' (a degree of laughter and innuendoes about ambulance control then proceeded to entertain them) for the rest of the journey back to station.

Taken from my fieldnotes (18/06/2013).

The enthusiasm and energy to which crews allocated to meal break avoidance and finishing their shift on time (off job) was significant. These somewhat deviant practices create a firmer foundation for students to be drawn into the subculture of the ambulance service. To a degree, this type of practice can also be seen in the work of Metz (1981), Mannon (1992), Corman (2017), and Palmer (1989) and, to some extent, in the work of McCann et al. (2013) and Wankhade and Mackway-Jones (2015). I found little, if any, evidence of change, as this practice was deeply embedded in the ambulance crews I was working with. We needed to understand how and why students were so readily drawn into this way of working, which is examined further in Chapter 6.

The final section in this chapter on paramedic professional identity explores the notion of dark humour (commonly known as black humour). The concept of black humour is often used by emergency personnel as a form of stress relief. There is a plethora of literature supporting this notion, such as Scott's (2007) work, which suggests emergency personnel need black humour to escape from the horrors of distressing and horrific incidents they encounter. Whilst obtaining our fieldnotes, I was often surprised by the use of the term black humour by students and experienced paramedics, although black humour is often used by the emergency service personnel to express their feelings following horrific sights and situations using jokes and innuendo. I found little, if any, use of black humour in response to horrific or tragic events. Our findings suggest that the notion of black humour was used more commonly as a means to justify and accord with more mundane non-traumatic events. The next section of this chapter examines this phenomenon and seeks to understand how and where black humour potentially fits within the data.

### 5.9.4 Black humour

At times, the notion of black humour became substituted for what could be perceived as cynical unprofessional behaviour or misconduct (HCPC, 2016). Somewhere amid all the formal university classroom development, student paramedics learn about the diverse group of individuals whom students will meet and treat, along with the social phenomena and cultures that the diverse group of people represent. The use of humour by healthcare professionals is acknowledged within the literature (McCreaddie & Wiggins, 2008), although this is in the context of traumatic events, as already identified. Our data, however, found both experienced paramedics and student paramedics would sometimes use derogatory and offensive language when referring to patients or members of the public. When challenged, the response from paramedics and students would often bracket these types of remarks as black humour, as a substitute for what we believe may have been a form of racism, and to justify the use of strong language, or simply as a purposeful illustration of unprofessional behaviour. In the following, we provide an example taken from the fieldnotes to help illustrate this.

> I was surprised and disappointed how Jane, the student appeared to agree with Mark, the paramedic when Mark voiced his opinion of the call we were attending. Both Jane and Mark agreed that we were going to a call that would be a 'load of old shit'. This will be some old 'alcoh' (alcoholic) depicting the call as a waste of fucking time. Then continuing to imply that paramedics should be able to undertake euthanasia! (Although I took this to be a figure of speech, rather than a literal intent.
> Taken from my fieldnotes (20/08/2013).

Rowe and Regehr (2010: 1) suggest, where stressful life-and-death situations occur, 'individuals would use black humour as a method of venting their feelings, eliciting social support through the development of group cohesion, and distancing themselves from a situation, ensuring that they can act effectively'. The following two observations provide an indication of where perceived black humour was exhibited by crews, which may not conform to the accepted understanding of the term.

> I am with the student (Peter) and a very experienced paramedic (Paul). I understand from Peter that Paul is perceived to be a 'dinosaur' (old timer), although Peter tells me he is okay! We attended a call to a

collapse and on arrival found a large obese female patient who had fallen off the commode. Both Peter and Paul worked well treating the patient and we, (I assisted), got the patient back into bed, as she had no apparent injuries. Although both Peter and Paul were very polite and kind to the patient. The post event conversation in the ambulance was very different, often referring to the patient as a smelly Lardy, (slang for someone who is obese), and claiming that she had eaten too many pies (football slang for obese people) (25/02/2013). I could not comprehend how this could be presented as black humour!

Taken from my fieldnotes (25/02/2013).

Whilst returning from our last call Tim, the paramedic spoke about how these people (the last patient) are a pain in the arse, referring to them as 'rag heads' a term I had heard whilst collecting data in the ambulance service when referring to people from either the Sikh or Asian community (The patient was of Indian origin). Although fortunately Caroline, the student didn't appear to engage with this dialogue (08/05/2013).

Taken from my fieldnotes (08/05/2013).

The following quotation taken from an interview of Mizrahi (1986) with a medical student helps lay out how the cynical views of other healthcare professionals may change over time:

When I was a brand-new third year medical student, I saw residents and interns joking about patients and I said I'll never do that . . .' I'm more cynical now. . . . I've definitely changed. . . . It's common for us to sit around clinic at the end of the day and ask, 'Well how many "pounds" did you see today?' and you talk about a two-ton and a four-ton clinic because I have at least two dozen women that weigh over 3000 pounds apiece.

(Mizrahi, 1986: 228)

We argue that this is not black humour, but a way in which practitioners became conditioned to talk about patients (punters) with other colleagues.

Whilst out on a night shift with the student (Tom) and paramedic (Sonia), I asked them both about their experiences of the 'watch-room' banter. I was trying to understand what they experienced and how they perceived the language and actions often associated with the watch-room environment. Both Tom and Sonia spoke about black humour, as a way of de-stressing, although often there was little if any evidence of correlation to actual events with that of subsequent behaviour. I challenged them on various racial and sexual comments, which were so often heard in this environment, both agreed this was unacceptable, yet believed it was still part of black humour.

Taken from my fieldnotes (10/03/2013).

Palmer (1983) highlights the unique and colourful use of terms described by crews when confronted with such devastating and grotesque and distressing events. I can recall terms such as. 'crispy critter' to describe someone who has burned to death, 'veggie' for an individual who has sustained a severe head injury (brain injury), and 'greenie' for a decomposing body. Scott's (2007) work refers to these although a subtle change in linguistics by the UK paramedics, who use terms such as 'stiff', denoting a person who has been deceased for some considerable time, or 'goner' for someone who has recently died. Charman (2013) suggests there is clearly a place to be found for black humour in emergency services work, to aid the de-stressing process, cope with the enormity of the situation, form bonds with each other, and to reinforce the group's values. This allows them to continue with their often demanding and unpredictable work. We accept that there may be a time when it becomes necessary to suspend professional behaviour in order to cope with the difficulties of dealing with discomforting events, as identified in the work of Scott (2007). However, what we found was not necessarily black humour but a way in which both experienced paramedics and students deal with day-to-day events, as also found in the work of Tangherlini (2000), Metz (1981), Palmer (1989), and Mannon (1992). This is a form of behaviour not expected nor warranted from healthcare professionals. The use of perverse and at times foul language to depict certain categories of people (patients) should not be confused with the accepted concept of black humour as a coping mechanism. Paramedics have a duty, responsibility, and an expectation to act with dignity and respect to patients (HCPC, 2019; COP, 2015). This was not always apparent from the findings.

Weaving a fabric of moral meaning into the day-to-day work of paramedics is somewhat challenging, as the paramedics' role is often multi-faceted, at times acting like a social worker, a police officer, a support worker, a teacher, and ultimately a carer (COP, 2019). The literature refers to black humour as being associated with the notion of death and dying and not superficial events which paramedics deal with daily, such as homeless people, the elderly, obese patient, alcohol-dependent patient, drug-addicted patient, and mentally ill patient. These categories of patients are amongst the most fragile and disparate group within society, which make up the majority of paramedics' workload. They require a caring and empathic approach to manage their often-complex medical needs. This is an important point which is highlighted within the data and examined further in Chapter 6, as the practice of using black humour to disguise poor behaviour of vulnerable distressed patients appeared widespread across many sections of data, both as discreet and overt presentations within the subculture, which we believe is unacceptable in today's modern NHS ambulance services.

This section of the chapter has explored issues which we have bracketed under the theme of paramedic professional identity, a strong and credible characteristic emerging from the data. We summarise our findings of professional identity, as that of meal break avoidance, off job, black humour, vandalism, and misconduct. The next section of this paragraph looks at institutionalisation and where this theme fits within the plethora of data. We use the term institutionalisation to capture the rigidity of university curricula, along with the bureaucratic nature of ambulance services. In doing so, we draw on our data to explore the relationship between university education and paramedic practice in helping to inform and further understand the student paramedic's practice experience.

### 5.9.5 Institutionalisation

The institutional influence here is to describe formal organisations and institutions, such as higher education institutions, the NHS, and the paramedic profession, along with other healthcare professions who have agency and, in a number of cases, hierarchical power structures and relations, which Lipsky (2010) relates to street-level bureaucracy, whilst institutionalisation refers to the 'action of establishing something as a convention or norm in an organisation or culture' (Stevenson 2002: 364). Our work explores the relationship embedded within the organisational culture of the ambulance service and provides examples of the mistrust and interplay between managers and crew staff. This is an important fundamental tenant of the practice setting as it provides a backdrop to inform the theme of institutionalisation. There were tensions between crew staff and students directed at the management of the organisation which needed to be understood, whilst Wankhade et al. (2018) indicate the striking similarities between the management style of all three emergency services, police, fire, and ambulance. The following extracts provide an indication of the distrust and resentment between front-line paramedic crews and managers.

---

This was my first of two weekend shifts and straightaway Pat, the experienced paramedic, not the student, stated why she thinks management are 'crap' (25/05/2013).

Taken from my fieldnotes (25/05/2013).

> Within the first 30 minutes of the shift, whilst the student and I were checking the vehicle, Pat constantly complained about the management of the Global City Ambulance Service, stating that: 'they are only interested in response times and "running you"' (Putting you on a disciplinary hearing) (25/05/2013).

The following section illustrates how this debate continued to be enacted out.

> Pat again spoke about the attitude of management and of the regulator, the Health Professions Council (HPC), now the Health and Care Professions Council (HCPC), suggesting they only want to report paramedics and to discipline those who do wrong. 'Response times and complaints are all they are interested in' (25/05/2013).
>    Taken from my fieldnotes (25/05/2013)

These sentiments were echoed by the students who subsequently voiced his concerns.

> The student (Mark), suggested that we (paramedics) shouldn't be regulated, seeking some reassurance from his paramedic colleague Pat, Mark added 'the poxy ambulance service always want to report you to the HPC, and they only want to strike you off the register, you know, get rid of you for the slightest thing, like complaining about how you spoke to someone, regardless of the person being a fucking pain the arse' (25/05/2013).
>    Taken from my fieldnotes (25/05/2013).

The views of Mark and Pat are interesting as they want to find agreement with each other's viewpoint. We needed to understand what was happening here. Lave and Wenger (1991) liken this kind of behaviour in the practice setting as a desire to belong to the community. This interaction supports previous examples of the fieldnotes where students are drawn into friendships with co-workers and mentors, regardless of the relationship being positive or negative. As Jordan (1989) claims, 'It's all about acceptance into the community'. The role of the paramedic is to attend, treat, and generally assist patients, some of whom may be difficult to assist for a variety of reasons, such as physical discomfort and/or pain, psychiatric conditions, some medical conditions such as a diabetic hypoglycaemic episode or fitting due to epilepsy, and intoxication or drug use, all of which can initiate sometimes aggressive and/or abusive behaviour from the patient (Moukaddam et al., 2015). The frustration from both the practitioner and student, along with the distrust of the ambulance service, depicts a sense of despair and frustration, a catalyst for debate amongst practitioners, as this position appears endemic within the service, as also seen in the work of Wankhade (2018). Arguably, the perceived unfairness in pay and conditions adds to the resentment and lack of trust with management by crew staff. This was evident in the observational fieldnotes taken on 02–05–13, which is illustrated here.

> After our first call, whilst at the hospital, we spoke about the amount of overtime being paid currently by the ambulance service (double time at weekends in addition to £120 attendance money). Although this attendance money would be withdrawn if the person (paramedic) was off sick within the same month. This caused much debate between (Mick) the student and (Andy) the paramedic, as Andy felt he was being discriminated against, as he worked reduced hours and was not entitled to this money. Both Mick and Andy continued to debate the 'perceived' unfairness of the pay-outs, both thought it unfair that the attendance allowance should be withdrawn if the person has any sickness within that month (02/05/2013).
>
> Taken from my fieldnotes (02/05/2013).

> Talking with (Sam) the paramedic, who added, 'the pay is okay when overtime payments are there, but that's not guaranteed and we work our balls off for what we get. I can't believe we (paramedics) are still on band five' (14/06/2013). (Band five refers to the National Agenda for Change (AFC), National NHS pay banding which equates to pay in the region of £20,000 to £30,000 per annum. To give some context to the banding, Nurses are generally paid a band six, or above, as are Physiotherapists which equates to a pay banding around 30,000 to 40,000. (14/04/2014).
>
> Taken from my fieldnotes (14/06/2013).

At the same time NHS ambulance services are working in a resource-starved environment, where the requirement to deliver prompt, appropriate, proportionate care to those who require their services (patients) is limited and stretched

'To be quite honest John (researcher), I am sick and tired of it. They (ambulance service) want us to work for them when we graduate but treat us like dirt as students. I won't be applying to this shower; I am going back home to Andover and work for them. They can't be any worse than this bunch' (13/05/2013 student William).

(The term 'shower' is used as jargon to illustrate the student's dissatisfaction and disappointment of the ambulance service).

Taken from my fieldnotes (13/05/2013).

There was a deep-rooted mistrust and dislike of ambulance control from experienced crews and students alike. Ambulance control have the responsibility of dispatching the response to the call as prescribed by the nature and extent of the 999 emergency call received within the control centre. This can consist of a fast response motorcar, motorcycle unit, cycle unit, air ambulance, and double crewed ambulance. This is how crews receive their calls from the ambulance dispatch centre. Consequently, it is central ambulance control who dictate the crews' workload, meal breaks, and, to a degree, their finishing times. This is important as it forms another key component of the subtle hidden curriculum in which students learn for themselves. To understand this, Lipsky, McCall, Wray and Lord, and Lave and Wenger offer some insight. Lipsky (2010) found people who work within these rigid intentional structures have a desire to 'fit in' to the organisation, not wanting to encounter negative attention, rather give a positive image. Lave and Wenger's (1991) work reviews the relationship between the Master, with that of the trainee apprentice, not wishing to upset the Master, but to do as they are told. Students mimic their role as full participants of the community rather than novices or peripheral participants. Students want to be central to their community of practice, rather than being peripheral in the practice setting, which McCall et al.'s (2009) work also illustrates. This has significant implications, both for the student and the profession. These tensions are explored later in Chapter 6 to help contextualise the emerging themes. The following examples help provide some initial context to this.

Already within the conversation there appeared to be distrust and disappointment with ambulance control, especially when ambulance control called the station to ask whether the ambulance from the previous night shift had returned as they (ambulance control) were holding an emergency call for us (the early turn) (06/04/2013).

Taken from my fieldnotes (06/04/2013).

Our first call is at 15:02 hours, just 2 min after starting duty, both student (Rees) and paramedic (Nigel) then complain about receiving the call whilst they are still checking the ambulance, I can sense their frustration as we have only just started the shift and need to get the vehicle ready and prepared. There appears to be general moans and groans about the control centre and the problems in allocating calls (12/04/2013).

Taken from my fieldnotes (12/04/2013).

We were able to sympathise with ambulance control, as they were also pressurised in meeting their targets. The following extract from a media broadcast provides some insight of the volume of work received by one ambulance control centre and the enormity of the task whilst working within a fragile infrastructure.

ambulance system failure 'might have led to patient death'. The London Ambulance Service are investigating whether computer failure early on New Year's Day may have contributed to the death of a patient. A Crew member remarks, 'we went from running a service to running a shamble's, people couldn't get ambulances. People couldn't get help'. They were waiting and waiting and waiting. For five hours, call-takers had to process every incident with pen and paper, and control room staff were limited to using radios to track and assign response units (ambulances).

(Ironmonger, 2017)

The extent to which the theme of institutionalisation informs this work depicts a somewhat restricted authoritarian organisation. Ambulance crews and students appear to be working within bureaucratic and often antiquated management systems. Modern technology has helped assist the operational arm of the ambulance service to deliver better healthcare. However, the day-to-day management of the organisation remains static and stagnant. For any significant change to occur, McCann et al. (2013) suggest that the cultural position of the organisation needs to shift. We explore this further in Chapter 6.

This section of the chapter has illustrated how the quasi-military nature of the ambulance service can influence and impact how people working within the organisation perceive those charged with managing and running the organisation. We found a deep mistrust and dislike from those on the front-line (paramedics) responsible for delivering the face-to-face service, with that of the bureaucratic organisational control placed over the paramedics by managers, like that of McCann et al.'s (2013) findings.

*5.9.6 Summary*

To summarise this chapter, our findings show three coexistent themes, consisting of paramedic work experience, institutionalisation, and paramedic professional identity. Each of these themes gave rise to certain working practices in which the students found themselves involved. As a result, a degree of enculturation took place which was informed by a hidden curriculum, which Andarvazh et al. (2017) infer are the unofficial, the unwritten, and often unintended lessons, values, and perspectives which students learn whilst in the practice setting. Furthermore, these practices lead to a form of pedagogy which students are neither informed of, nor aware of, and therefore contribute to the students' learning and development as paramedics.

The findings have drawn on various sources of evidence to help position and expose some of this hidden curriculum embedded within the subculture of an inner-city metropolitan NHS ambulance service trust. This illustrates how these findings are an integral part of a professional social structure within a working environment which spans formal authoritarian (quasi-military) control, with a constrained (front-line) workforce.

The proceeding chapter will explore the implications for the role of paramedics. It will argue how the subculture of the ambulance service contributes to the student's epistemological development in identifying the precise nature of student enculturation and their journey, from classroom learning to situational understandings within a hidden curriculum which informs their pedagogy. It will argue that, for any significant change to occur, work experiences and professional identity, along with the stringent structurally confined organisation, such as the ambulance service (Devenish, 2014; Donaghy, 2011; Wankhade & Brinkman, 2014; Reynolds, 2004; O'Meara, 2011; Givati et al., 2018), require significant change at both the macro (professional) level and micro (individual) level.

## References

Andarvazh, R. M., Afshar, L. & Yazdani, S. (2017) 'Hidden curriculum: An analytical definition', *Journal of Medical Education*, 16(4), pp. 198–207.

Armitage, E. (2010) 'Role of paramedic mentors in an evolving profession', *Journal of Paramedic Practice*, 2(1), pp. 26–31.

Association of Ambulance Chief Executives (AACE). (2016) https://aace.org.uk

Becker, H. (1963) *Outsiders: Studies in the Sociology of Deviance*. New York: The Free Press.

Becker, H. (1964) *The Other Side: Perspectives on Deviance*. New York: The Free Press.

Becker, H. (1970) *Sociological Work: Methods and Substance*. London/New York: Routledge, p. 133.

Bell, A. (2010) 'The subculture concept: A genealogy', in S. G. Shoham, P. Knepper & M. Kett (Eds.), *International Handbook of Criminology*. Boca Raton, FL: CRC Press.

Boychuck Duchscher, E. J. & Cowin, S. L. (2004) 'The experience of marginalisation in new nursing graduates', *Nursing Outlook*, 52(6), pp. 289–296.

Breen, J. L. (2007) 'The researcher "in the middle": Negotiating the insider/outsider dichotomy', *The Australian Community Psychologist*, 19(1).

Burgess, A. (2010) 'The use of space-time to construct identify and context', *Ethnography and Education*, 5(1), pp. 17–31.

Burt, C. (1925) *The Sub-Normal School Child: The Young Delinquent*. London: University of London Press Ltd.

Care Quality Commission. (2015) https://www.cqc.org.uk/sites/default/files/20160721_annualreport_2015-16.pdf

Charman, S. (2013) 'Sharing a laugh', *International Journal of Sociology and Social Policy*, 33(3/4), pp. 152–166.

College of Paramedics – Curriculum Guidance. (2015) https://nasemso.org/wp-content/uploads/UKParamedic_Curriculum_Guidance_2015.pdf

College of Paramedic's Curriculum Guidance Framework. (2019) https://collegeof-paramedics.co.uk/?gclid=Cj0KCQjwqs6lBhCxARIsAG8YcDhZ5NQeSilXkhny3r CZar2RjVxkoY--4ecNyLV8wg-3THvxjpoD0R0aAqrfEALw_wcB

Corman, K. M. (2017) *Paramedics On and Off the Streets-Emergency Medical Services in the Age of Technological Governance*. Toronto/Buffalo/London: University of Toronto Press.

Cowin, L. S. & Hengstberger-Sims, C. (2004) 'New graduate nurse self-concept and retention: A longitudinal survey', *International Journal of Nursing Studies*, 43, pp. 59–70.

Coyne, I., Craig, J. & Smith-Lee Chong, P. (2004) 'Workplace bullying in a group context', *British Journal of Guidance & Counselling*, 32(3), pp. 301–317.

Devenish, A. S. (2014) 'Experiences in becoming a Paramedic: A qualitative study examining the university qualified paramedics', *Creative Education*, 7(6), pp. 786–801.

Devenish, A. S., Clark, M. J. & Fleming, M. L. (2016) 'Experience in becoming a paramedic: The professionalisation of university qualified paramedics', *Creative Education*, 7(7).

Donaghy, J. (2010) 'Equipping the student for the workplace changes in paramedic education', *Journal of Paramedic Practice*, 2(11), pp. 524–528.

Donaghy, J. (2011) 'Is regulation a necessary evil?', *Journal of Paramedic Practice*, 3(3), p. 109.

Furber, R. (2008) *Curriculum Guidance & Competency Framework Document*, 2nd ed. Bridgwater: College of Paramedics, p. 2.

Givati, A., Markham, C. & Street, K. (2018) 'The bargaining of professionalism in emergency care practice: NHS paramedics and higher education', *Advances in Health Science Education*, 23, p. 353.

Gray, A. & Harrison, S. (2004), *Governing Medicine: Theory and Practice*. Buckingham/new York: Open University Press.

Grusec, J. E. & Hastings, P. D. (2015) *Handbook of Socialization: Theory and Research,* 3rd ed. New York/London: Guildford Press.

Health and Care Professions Council (HCPC). (2016) *Health Care Professions Council – Social Work*. http://www.hcpc-uk.org/aboutregistration/professions/index.asp?id=18#profDetails (Accessed 2nd February 2016).

Hafferty, J. W. & O'Donnell, J. F. (2014) *Introduction: The Hidden Curriculum – A Focus on Learning and Closing the Gap, Medical Teacher*. Hanover/New England: Health Professional Education, Dartmouth College Press.

Health and Care Professions Council (HCPC). (2019) *Protecting the Public Promoting Professionalism Fitness to Practise*. Annual Report.

Ironmonger, J. (2017) 'British Broadcasting Corporation (BBC) news report', *News*, 6 January 2017. London, UK.

Jordan, B. (1989) 'Cosmopolitical obstetrics: Some insights from the training of traditional midwives', *Social Science and Medicine*, 28(9), pp. 925–944.

Kline, R., Naqvi, H., Razaq, S. & Wilhelm, R. (2017) *NHS workforce race equality standard. 2016 Data analysis report for NHS Trusts*. United Kingdom NHS. https://www.england.nhs.uk/wp-content/uploads/2017/03/workforce-race-equality-standard-data-report-2016.pdf

Lave, J. & Wenger, E. (1991) *Situated Learning: Legitimate Peripheral Participation*. Cambridge/New York/Melbourne/Madrid/Cape Town/: Cambridge University Press.

Lipsky, M. (2010) *Street-Level Bureaucracy Dilemmas of the Individual in Public Services*. New York: Russel Sage Foundation.

Lovegrove, M. & Davis, J. (2013) *Paramedic Evidence-Based Education Project (PEEP): End of Study Report*. Buckinghamshire: Allied Health Solutions/Buckinghamshire New University.

Mannon, M. J. (1992) *Emergency Encounters – EMTs and Their Work*. Boston, MA: Jones and Bartlett.

Martimianakis, M. A., Maniate, J. M. & Hodges, B. D. (2009) 'Sociological interpretations of professionalism', *Medical Education*, 43(9), pp. 829–837.

McCall, L., Wray, N. & Lord, B. (2009) 'Factors affecting the education of pre-employment paramedic students during the clinical practicum', *Journal of Emergency Primary Health Care*, 7(4).

McCann, L., Granter, E., Hyde, P. & Hassard, J. (2013) 'Still blue-collar after all these years? An ethnography of the professionalisation of emergency work', *Journal of Management Studies*, 50(5), pp. 750–774.

McCreaddie, M. & Wiggins, S. (2008) 'The purpose and function of humour in health, health care and nursing: A narrative review', *Journal of Advanced Nursing*, 61(6), pp. 584–594. https://doi.org/10.1111/j.1365-2648.2007.04548

McLaughlin, H., Ugreen, C. & Blackstone, A. (2012) 'Sexual harassment, workplace, authority, and the paradox of power', *American Sociological*, 77(40), pp. 625–647.

McNamee, S. & Glasser, M. (1987–1988) 'The power concept in sociology: A theoretical Assessment', *Humboldt Journal of Social Relations*, 15(1) (Fall/Winter 1987–88), p. 79.

Metz, L. D. (1981) *Running Hot-Structure and Stress in Ambulance Work*, 1st ed. Edited by L. D. Metz. Cambridge, MA: Abt Books.

Mizrahi, T. (1986) *Getting Rid of Patients: Contradictions in the Socialization of Physicians*. New Brunswick, NJ: Rutgers University Press.

Moukaddam, N., AufderHeide, E., Flores, A. & Tucci, V. (2015) 'Shift, interrupted: Strategies for managing difficult patients including those with personality disorders and somatic symptoms in the emergency department', *Emergency Medical Clinician*, 33, pp. 797–810.

Mowforth, G. (1999) 'Power and nursing practice', *Sociology and Nursing Practice Series*, 3.

Mulder, H., ter Braak, E., Chen, H. C. & Cate, O. T. (2019) 'Addressing the hidden curriculum in the clinical workplace: A practical tool for trainees and faculty', *Medical Teacher*, 41(1), pp. 36–43. https://doi.org/10.1080/0142159X.2018.1436760

O'Meara, P. (2011) 'So how can we frame our identity?', *Journal of Paramedic Prac-*
   *tice.* paramedicpractice.com.
Palmer, E. (1983) ' "Trauma Junkie" and street work: Occupational behaviour of
   paramedics and emergency medical technicians', *Journal of Contemporary Ethnog-*
   *raphy, Urban Life* (2), pp. 162–183.
Palmer, E. (1989) 'Paramedic performance', *Sociological Spectrum*, 9, pp. 211–225.
Public   Health   England.   (2020)   https://www.gov.uk/government/organisations/
   public-health-england/about
Reynolds, L. (2004) 'Is prehospital care really a profession', *Journal of Emergency
   Primary Health Care*, 2.
Rowe, A. & Regehr, C. (2010) 'Whatever gets you through today: An examination
   of cynical humour among emergency service professionals', *Journal of Loss and
   Trauma. International Perspectives on Stress and Coping*, 15(5).
Scott, T. (2007) 'Expression of humour by emergency personnel involved in sudden
   death work', *Mortality*, 12(4), pp. 350–364.
Sharar, B. (2016) *Emergent Pedagogy in England: A Critical Realist Study of
   Structure-Agency Interactions in Higher Education*. London/New York: Routledge.
Shprakh, V., Gorbacheva, S. & Golubchikova, M. (2019) 'Development of additional
   professional medical education organisation in accordance with the principles of
   quality management', *Medical University*, 2(2).
Stevenson, A. (2002) *Concise Oxford English Dictionary*, 2nd ed rev. Oxford: Oxford
   University Press.
Tangherlini, R. T. (2000) 'Heroes and lies: Storytelling tactics among paramedics',
   *The Folklore Society*. Routledge Journals.
van der Gaag, A. & Donaghy, J. (2013) 'Paramedics and professionalism: Looking
   back and looking forwards', *Journal of Paramedic Practice*. Mark Allen Group,
   5(1), pp. 8–10.
Wankhade, P. (2015) 'Different cultures of management and their relationships with
   organisational performance: Evidence from the UK ambulance service', *Public
   Money & Management*, pp. 381–388.
Wankhade, P. (2018) 'The crisis in NHS ambulance services in the UK: Let's deal with
   the 'elephants in the room'!', *Ambulance Today*, 15(1), pp. 13–17.
Wankhade, P. & Brinkman, J. (2014) 'The negative consequences of cultural man-
   agement: Evidence from a UK ambulance service', *International Journal of Public
   Sector Management*, 27(1), pp. 2–25.
Wankhade, P., McCann, L. & Murphy, P. (2018) *Management Critical Perspec-
   tives on the Management and Organization of Emergency Services*. New York:
   Routledge.
Wankhade, P. & Mackway-Jones, K. (2015) *Understanding the Management of
   Ambulance Services Ambulance Services: Leadership and Management Perspec-
   tives*. Cham/Heidelberg/New Yor/Dordrecht/London: Springer.
Weber, M. (1968) *Economy and Society: An Outline of Interpretive Sociology*.
   Edited by G. Roth & C. Wittich (translations by various authors). New York:
   Bedminster.
Williams, B. (2005) 'Case based learning – A review of the literature: Is there scope
   for this educational paradigm in prehospital education?', *Emergency Medical Jour-
   nal Online*, 22, pp. 577–581.

Willis, E., Williams, B., Brightwell, R., O'Meara, P. & Pointon, T. (2010) 'Road-ready paramedics and the supporting sciences curriculum', *Focus on Health Professional Education: A Multi-Disciplinary Journal*, 11(2), pp. 1–13.

Zapf, D. & Einarsen, S. (2003) *Individual Antecedents of Bullying. Bullying and Emotional Abuse in the Workplace: International Perspective in Research and Practice*. London/New York: Taylor & Francis.

# 6 Discussion

## 6.1 Introduction

In this chapter, we outline the theoretical framework used to structure the discussion. This draws on the concepts of the formal and informal phases of paramedic education, subculture, and subsequent hidden curriculum which gives rise to it. Furthermore, models of enculturation are reviewed (Jackson, 1968; Brewer, 2000; McCann et al., 2013; Wankhade & Mackway-Jones, 2015), whilst Schein's (1985) model of organisational culture, along with Lave and Wenger's (1991 and Wenger's (1998) use of communities of practice, is justified over more recent models that expand on the original work of Lave and Wenger, such as Boychuk Duchscher and Cowin's (2004) concept of marginalisation.

By using an ethnography, this thesis investigated the enculturation of student paramedics by drawing on the aforementioned theoretical models with a view to identifying the processes by which students experience the clinical workplace in the context of university paramedic education (van Maanen, 2011). We recognise the aspects of enculturation are relevant to teaching, nursing, and medicine, as also seen in the work of Jackson (1968), Henderson (2011), Rankin and Campbell (2006), Cant and Higgs (1999), and Becker et al. (1961). We draw on relevant research literature in paramedic training, schools, medical socialisation, and nurse education to support our findings.

The findings found in Chapter 5 sit within an overarching organisational (parent) culture which is depicted within the ambulance service. Yet our findings also illustrate the existence of an entrenched subculture, embedded within the National Health Service (NHS) ambulance trust where the study was conducted. This subculture shapes and informs a hidden curriculum giving rise to a specific type of student learning. We would also argue that this subculture is not unique to one particular NHS ambulance trust, rather these findings can reasonably be looked upon as widespread and embedded with other trusts. We launch this viewpoint from a position of experience and various derogatory media reports, along with the fitness to practice (FTP) cases referred to the regulator. Overall, the data illustrated culturally

DOI: 10.4324/9781032721408-6

different ideas and expectations of the working environment to that expected by the academic community, along with the professional and regulatory bodies. There were differences in the pedagogic and professional context of the workplace setting which paramedic students struggled to adapt to and which impinged on the application of learning and impeded workplace pedagogy. Hafler et al. (2011) suggest medical student literature has broadly found the importance of differentiating between the formal-explicit and hidden-tacit dimensions of the clinician education process. The hidden curriculum refers to cultural norms which can be conveyed but not openly acknowledged.

We discuss how the three dominate themes drawn out of the data provide a scaffold to help explore the paramedic students' enculturation into the working environment of the ambulance service which gives rise to the cultural norms and traditions ingrained within a very structured and autocratic institution, as inferred in the work of McCann et al. (2013). We also set out to understand how and why this ingrained subculture and subsequent hidden curriculum became so prominent and dominant throughout the findings.

In the next section of the chapter, we discuss the relationship between the research findings and the wider theoretical concepts which help strengthen and underpin this work. Furthermore, the chapter defines the process of enculturation into the working environment. It concludes with the research findings whilst drawing out implications for practice.

## 6.2 The relationship of data to a conceptual framework

We were mindful of Jackson's (1968) study on school children which popularised the term hidden curriculum. Conducting intensive observations of school children in the classroom, Jackson noted that the day-to-day conduct of schooling appeared to be a strong influence on children's values and beliefs which Bain (1985: 145), reviewing Jackson's work, found that 'students learned patience, acceptance of impersonal prescriptive authority and distinctions between work and play'. In addition, students learned to conform to institutional expectations. The work highlights the impact of the hidden curriculum and questions whether the patterns and customs of schooling are functional or dysfunctional, harmful, or harmless. We needed to understand the hidden curriculum, as this is a key finding drawn from the data. To do this we looked at the work of Giroux and Penna (2012: ii) who state that hidden curriculum's 'covert patterns of socialisation, may prepare students to function in the existing workplace and in other political spheres'. They argue that social processes of school provide specific meaning to the term 'hidden curriculum'. The work of Hafferty (1998) found a deep-rooted hidden curriculum is evident within medical education, suggesting that what is often taught in the formal setting of the classroom has little resemblance to what occurs in the busy turbulent clinical setting. Contextualising the concept in medical education by arguing that connections exist between group membership, socialisation, institutional authority, and patterns of perception, which as Hafferty implies, resonates with the hidden curriculum in medical education. Therefore, students are drawn into a very different form of learning in the workplace, to that which is taught in the university.

Becker et al. (1961) found medical students grouped together to form their own communities. These communities were subversive and aimed to survive the established rules and regulations of medical training and excessive workloads. Lave and Wenger (1991) believe learning is situated within the social context of the workplace, suggesting that knowledge is drawn from the workplace experience. Devenish (2014) discusses organisational socialisation theories to understand the possible socialisation of ambulance staff prior to undertaking paramedic education and training in universities. Consisting of three stages, the socialisation theory separates the pre-socialisation phase, the formal socialisation phase, and the post-formal socialisation phase. Devenish (2014) also found that academisation is not without its problems and concluded that:

> There can be conflict between older workers trained within the traditional model and younger workers educated within the universities. The paramedicine profession in Australia is still in the midst of the academisation process.
>
> (Devenish, 2014: 27)

We were drawn back to Schein's theory of organisational culture to reveal a structure which identifies the preconceptions of the public outside of the organisation, the taken-for-granted assumptions of the organisation and universities, and, lastly, what really goes on in the workplace. Our adaptation of Schein's (1985) model highlights the discord found between these three areas and provides an understanding to what we have unearthed in our findings. We then looked at Kramer's (1974) work, of post qualified (new) nurses who went through a short 'honey-moon period', as nurses felt wholly unready for the workplace, suggesting that they become focused solely on skills and routine mastery which Lave and Wenger (1991) identify in their work on apprenticeships, whilst Whitehead (2001) suggests newly qualified nurses have a different perspective of their role. This helped us identify certain areas with our findings, whilst also assimilating the relationship found in the skills-based approach to the learning situation.

To address the subculture and hidden curriculum, whilst understanding the social aspects in which this specific subculture is situated, we needed to understand social integration, as students attempt to gain acceptance into the community by forming relationships with their paramedic colleagues, sometimes attending work functions and events (Kramer, 1974). Although, just creating these relationships does not ensure students become comfortable, as students become suspicious and frustrated due to their unrealistic expectations based on their university education, which often depicts a different form of learning, to that experienced in the workplace. Kramer (1974) refers to this as being the 'moral outrage' phase, as students experience a paradox between the two learning environment. Considering this, we looked at Lave and Wenger's (1991) communities of practice. This enabled us to illustrate how and why paramedic students may unwittingly become an integral and inseparable part of the community in which they were exposed to in the ambulance workplace. Figure 6.1 helps to illustrate the various components of the learning process as depicted from Lave and Wenger's (1991) model of communities of practice. In the centre lies the integral involvement of practice and the experienced practitioners (old-timers), whilst the middle circle represents the various forms of learning, such as learning through engagement with other members of the workplace community, for instance interaction with colleagues and collaboration with other members of the learning environment, for example hospital staff, nurses, doctors, and other emergency service personnel. These help to shape and inform the learning, knowledge,

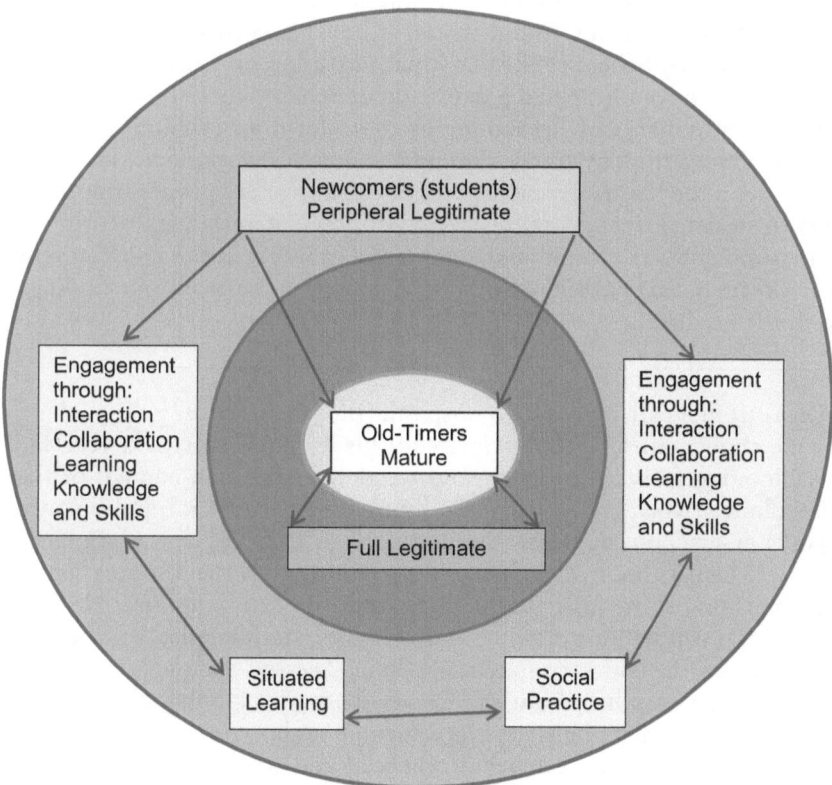

*Figure 6.1* Lave and Wenger's (1991) model depicting communities of practice.

and skills which the student acquires through this form of social interaction. As a result of this, students move from a position of being peripheral participants of the practice community to one of full legitimate participants as they learn the social practices and situated learning which are integral to the workplace. The student has now become a mature experienced practitioner (old-timer) through the concept of communities of practice. The figure helps depict the student journey, from newcomers to legitimate participants and depicts the social practice and situated learning which influences and shapes their workplace learning.

Considering the aforementioned discussion, an appreciation of how students become enculturated into the cultural surroundings is apparent, as they engage in the complex relationships of the workplace culture, as opposed to the culture prescribed within the university setting. The behaviours and cultural norms which the students move through to get to the centre are numerous and diverse, as students go about their day-to-day work placements. To try and answer this dichotomy, we looked at Schein's (1985) model of organisational culture along with any relationship to Lave and Wenger's (1991) communities of practice. By doing so we were able to unearth the comparisons found in our study between the cultural differences identified by Schein (1985) and that of studies on work placements. In Chapter 3, we have illustrated a depiction of Schein's model to help identify the three components of his model, as these form an essential part of the study, depicting the day-to-day 'goings on' of the workplace. The dichotomy between the theory-based aspects of the university programme and the ability of students to enact these aspects of practice in the 'real world' clinical environment was at best challenging and at worst impossible (Devenish, 2014; Corman, 2017). We provide an example taken from our findings to help illustrate this.

After our first call, on route to hospital, (Jim) the student, was speaking to me about returning to university for his last final year, next year. He was looking forward to it, he told me that he has had enough of the ambulance 'world'. Jim said how much he loved the job (ambulance work) at first, but as he has been treated so badly by the Ambulance Service, such as poor rotas, being messed around by the resource centre and finishing shifts late, that he now hates the 'stinking job'. He told me how much he likes dealing with patients, stating that, 'I still enjoy that side of the job very much, but being messed around so much is just crazy'. He spoke about the University students being placed onto 'X' relief rota which he states- 'is a fucking nightmare'. (X relief incorporates an additional number of unsocial and weekend working). He appeared so angry of the position (student paramedic), which he was once so proud of being accepted onto, proved to be so poor, due to the way the staff, especially students, were being treated. I asked if he felt that maybe the University could do something to support students, for example, speaking with the Ambulance Service. Jim replied, 'Well you know John, nothing will ever change that, the ambulance service has no career structure for staff or students and it appears that they really don't care about you, as long as you meet their targets' (Observational fieldnotes recorded on 07/12/2014 whilst in the ambulance travelling to hospital).

Students who dared to challenge the traditional accepted norms and the so-called 'banter' of the day-to-day work were ostracised from the working environment by the more experienced paramedics. Drawing on the students' experiences, we argue that the subculture identified from our findings can be related to Schein's (1985) pluralistic dimension of culture, which is defined as:

A model of organisational culture where the basic assumptions shape values and the values shape practices and behaviour, which is the visible part of culture.

Schein (1985: 17)

The work of McCann et al. (2013), helps illustrate the institutional culture within the ambulance service. McCann et al. (2013) found a rigid form of organisational culture existed, which could be considered as an authoritarian, quasi-military style service which restricts and detracts from the day-to-day operational demands experienced by those on the front-line, such as the experienced paramedics and student paramedics. To cope with this, our data shows paramedics develop their own unique observable patterns of behaviours, beliefs, and values which become implicit in shaping and reinforcing the subculture. These types of behaviour inform and shape the hidden curriculum, as recognised by Kelly (2006), Corman (2016), and Wankhade and Mackway-Jones (2015), and further supported by Hafferty's (1998) and Becker et al.'s (1961) work on medical education. Hafferty and O'Donnell's (2014) findings have some similarities, as they found students were following the largely unconscious beliefs and expectations which formed a deep and largely hidden subculture. Hafferty and O'Donnell (2014: 18) argue that 'faculties feel more comfortable reengineering the formal curriculum than they do redesigning the learning environments that make up, in this case medical school experiences.' Similar issues present themselves within the harsh, totalitarian structure of the ambulance service, which Wankhade and Mackway-Jones (2015) and McCann et al. (2013) also identify, as opposed to the relative academic freedom of university. One example of the rigid formal quasi-military style of the ambulance service is provided in the following, taken from our findings.

---

After one incident whist we were at the hospital handing over our patient, we were asked by an ambulance officer to try and call control as quickly as possible as they (ambulance control) were holding emergency calls and there were no other resources available. Both the experienced paramedic and student paramedic subsequently thought up a fictitious reason to return to station, rather than conform to the officer's instructions (Observational fieldnotes recorded on 05/12/2014 whilst waiting to handover patient at treetop hospital).

---

Whilst riding out with Paul the student and Tim the paramedic, I watched how Paul tried to listen to an elderly female's abdomen with his stethoscope (this would be normal practice that is taught at university for listening to bowel sounds etc). I was not overly surprised to hear Tim, the paramedic, announce that, 'we don't do all that old tosh around here Paul, just let's get the chair and go to hospital'. Paul, obliged and put his stethoscope back in his trouser pocket, whilst they put the patient in the carry chair (Observational fieldnotes recorded on 23/04/2014 whilst in the patient's house).

---

Similarly, Lipsky's (2010) work on public sector workers found that public housing officers and police officers often formed their own unique working subcultures, as opposed to the autocratic culture imposed by their respective organisations. Lipsky's work illustrates some examples of the organisational subcultures which exist independently to that of their (parent) organisational culture and which can lead to small work groups forming their own set of values and beliefs, similar to the work of Brown (2002), Martin and Siehl (1983), Sackman (1991), andBrewer (1991) suggest that if the parent culture is not sufficiently strong the subculture becomes predominant. This can lead to students becoming rooted into the day-to-day working practices. We link this back to how Paul, the student paramedic, tried to listen to an elderly female's abdominal (bowel) sounds yet was prevented from doing so by the more experienced (old-timer) paramedic. Crawford and Lok (1999) conclude from their study that the organisational subculture had a larger effect on organisational engagement than did the organisational (parent) culture.

Boychuck Duchscher (2009) found students can become 'emotionally terrified' and 'scared to death' when they go into the workplace in fear of being incompetent. Students become physically and mentally exhausted because of trying to meet the workplace expectations.

In this section, we have tried to unpack the relationship between Schein's (1985) model of organisational culture with that of our findings. We examine how Lave and Wenger's (1991) communities of practice offers an understanding of how and why students form unique, often subversive, communities of practice, whilst acknowledging other theoretical concepts which relate to similar aspects that have been identified in the findings. In the next section of the chapter, we lay out enculturation and illustrate how, because of forming unique communities of practice, students become enculturated into a specific subculture and hidden curriculum.

## 6.3 Enculturation

This ethnography draws on participant's interaction with the experienced paramedics, other medical staff, and patients/public. It is an ethnographic study, albeit one that took place at sporadic intervals between fulltime work, homelife, and occasional periods of leisure (holidays), rather than a continuous field study.

The study involved working with the students over many months to facilitate describing and interpreting the shared patterns of culture experienced by participants (Moore, 2000). However, this ethnography is not based on an institutional ethnography specifically (Campbell et al., 2015), although the very essence of observing people in the workplace over a prolonged period of time creates data which identifies and illustrates the real-life working practices and behaviours of student paramedics and experienced paramedics, similar to that found in the work of Crawford and Lok (1999). This is a central feature of ethnographic research whereby a variety of cultures may arise from the working environment.

Our ethnography gave rise to certain working practices in which the students found themselves drawn into. This process operated as a hidden curriculum, where the knowledge learned is historically, culturally, and situationally constituted within the practice setting, such as that supported by Lave and Wenger (1991). A hidden curriculum draws on the concept of curricula as a series of experiences which students go through. 'Lessons which are learned but not openly intended' (Martin & Siehl, 1983: 122), as Kelly (2006) implies, are responsible for some of the social roles which are learnt in this way, such as aspects of living and working. Hafferty and O'Donnell (2014) further suggest that learning in medical education takes place, to some degree, outside of the formal curriculum. Hafferty (1998) also infers that subcultures need particular exploration if we are to uncover the institution and workplace's hidden curricula. Although ill-defined, Jackson (1968) found the hidden curriculum is associated with the unintentional learning which occurs in the practice setting, which is in addition to any formal structured curriculum, such as that delivered at university. We found that this unintentional learning became evident in the workplace which informed and shaped students' pedagogy, as they became drawn into a subculture far removed from that envisaged by the university curriculum (Andarvazh et al., 2017). We reminded ourselves that participatory practices are however mutually constructed, as individuals decide if and how to enlist in and learn from these workplace practices (Billett, 2002). Students had little, if any, choice in these workplace practices, because failure to engage in them resulted in hostility and rejection from their community of practitioners.

Mulder et al. (2019) look at the hidden curriculum in the clinical workplace of a hospital and provide striking similarities to the paramedics' clinical workplace experiences. Mulder et al.'s (2019) work presents a practical method to facilitate reflection and consider the hidden curriculum by all those involved. Using a non-judgemental conceptual framework, they suggest early experiences of addressing the hidden curriculum can be beneficial. The following extract helps illustrate this.

> That much of what happens in the clinical environment is not prescribed nor foreseen in curriculum documents. Medical education literature uses the term hidden curriculum to refer to the set of implicit messages about values, norms and attitudes that learners infer from the behaviour of individual role models as well as from group dynamics, processes, rituals and structure.
>
> (Mulder et al., 2019: 1)

McCann et al.'s (2013) work found a perceived distrust and resentment in the ambulance service between management and front-line crew staff, which originates from the institutional context. Policy makers at both the macro (governmental) and micro (institutional) level become far removed from the realities of delivery and the often unrealistic and arbitrary restrictions and targets which drive the institutional processes. Lipsky (2010) refers to front-line practitioners as *street-level bureaucrats*, working face to face in public service. These street-level bureaucrats often form their own unique working practices and behaviours as a response to unreasonable and unrealistic targets and delivery of service. A consequence of which results in workers forming their own systems and traditions of working. We provide some examples here in which these forms of working practices and behaviours, as highlighted by Lipsky (2010), are evident in our findings.

- *Paramedics and students were constantly avoiding their official meal breaks to finish their rostered shift early and receive monetary remuneration* (as depicted in the fieldnotes and recorded whilst riding out with Tim, experienced paramedic and Paul, student paramedic (06/04/2013).

- *Crews would often report or create various vehicle (ambulance) defects to avoid a late emergency call when they were nearing the end of their shift* (as depicted in the fieldnotes whilst riding out with Trevor, experienced paramedic (13/04/2013).
- *Crews would generally try to manipulate their day-to-day work to remain local to their geographic location nearer to their ambulance station* (as depicted in the fieldnotes whilst riding out with Tony, experienced paramedic, and Sally, student paramedic (12/04/2013).

These working practices give rise to a complex web of sociocultural conditions which formed the very fabric of the placement setting.

We further acknowledge that some components of our data were collected several years ago, although we would argue that little, if any, significant change has occurred to address these issues. Students returning to university, following periods of clinical placement practice, still encounter cultures which are steeped in traditional ways of working, unacceptable behaviours, and lack of trust by managers, as those when the original data was collected.

Thornton and Nardi (1975) divide the informal and personal socialisation phases by defining roles as behavioural, attitudinal, and cognitive expectations. The passive phase appears to be reflective of the 'hidden curriculum' outlined by Hafferty and O'Donnell (2014), whilst the formal phase involves students immersing themselves in the culture. They observe and assimilate behaviours that support their progression, easing each other's social anxiety. In the personal socialisation phase, students begin to combine their previous preconceptions with the expectations of others within the profession. They seek to take on a new identity, which the work of Thornton and Nardi (1975) demonstrates. Students identify with the work culture during this phase, as they begin to engage with the banter and accepted norms and workplace practices which can comprise of a demanding, unpredictable, and challenging working environment. This can result in confusion and resentment by the students as they come to terms with the complexities of the paramedic workplace. We provide an illustration here, Figure 6.2, to help depict the complex structure in which students adapt to the practice setting.

The illustration shows the interrelating themes of pedagogy in the field. The large circle stands for the communities of practice which became a common thread throughout the research, as students became exposed to, and an integral part of, the practice community. The smaller circle represents the three themes, consisting of work experience, institutionalisation, and professional identity, which sit within the communities of practice and influence, and are influenced by tensions, represented by the arrows. Pedagogy is represented by the circle positioned within the central triangle, which is influenced by a hidden curriculum emerging from the entrenched subculture of the paramedic working environment.

During the enculturation process, students became anxious because of the work-based responsibilities (work experiences), combined with being

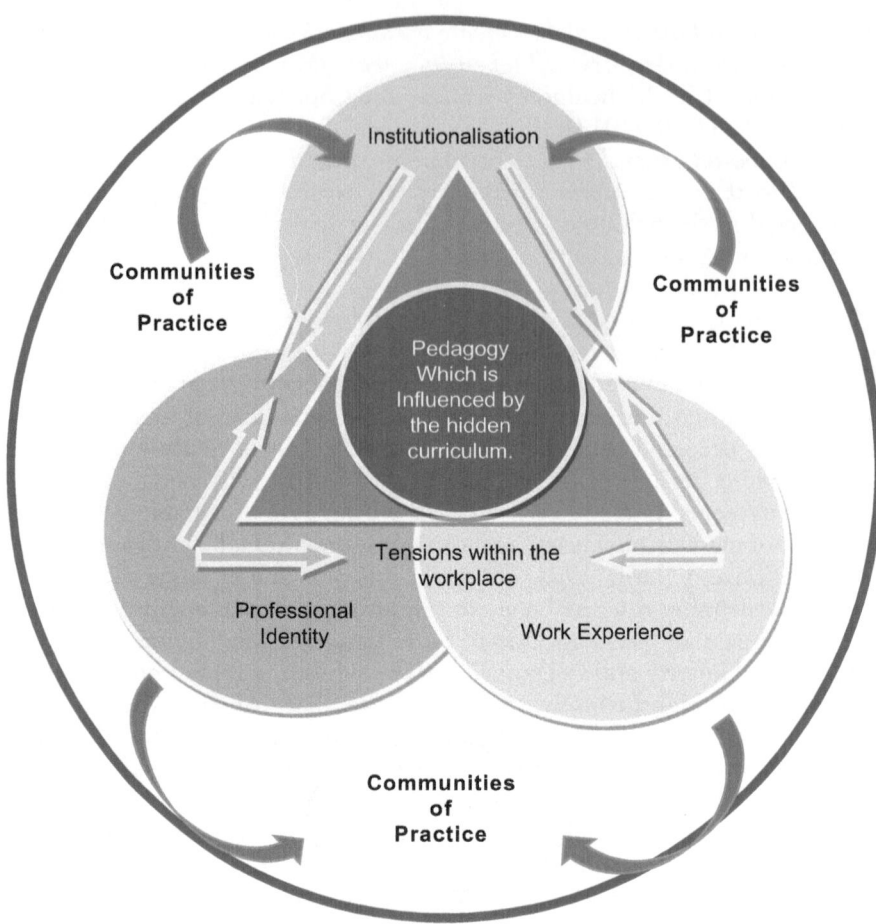

*Figure 6.2* Model of enculturation.

a student (professional identity), and fear of making mistakes and getting into trouble with their mentor or ambulance managers (institutionalisation). Kramer (1974) found that new nurses regard the experienced nurses to be judging them. Similarly, Boychuck Duchscher (2009) found students became under pressure to emulate work practices which prioritised ritualistic routines, as opposed to clinical interaction with patients. Students were concerned that their inexperience and lack of acceptance in the practice setting were compromised whilst trying to practise what they were taught by their educational institution, whilst assimilating the practices carried out in clinical practice. Boychuck Duchscher and Cowin's (2004) work sheds some light on this process, as they found that newly qualified nurses can experience a form of marginalisation in the workplace for some time. We found

Devenish's (2014) study is of particular interest, as university paramedic students encountered similar isolation and hostility in the paramedic workplace, as also identified by Boyle et al. (2008) and Lord (2009), as they transitioned from their academic studies to their workplace. This can create a form of marginalisation as students undergo the enculturation process.

In this section, we have illustrated how student enculturation emerged from the various components of the observational fieldnotes, interviews, and reflexive accounts. These interact with the theoretical literature such as Lave and Wenger's (1991) communities of practice which contribute to the theoretical framework of this research. In the next section, a particular form of pedagogy which occurred in the workplace is explored. This is one of the fundamental tenants of the work and one which gives rise to the enculturation of students due to the relationship with workplace learning.

## 6.4 Pedagogy

The emerging subtle pedagogy identified in our research often manifested itself as a discrete, yet powerful, learning experience whereby students became drawn into the traditional subculture of the working practices which subsequently enculturated them into the practice setting, which Hafferty and O'Donnell (2014), Burns (2002), Lave and Wenger (1991), and Devenish (2014) suggest is part of the socialisation process, as also seen in the work of van Maanen (2011) and Freire (1985) who imply this results in a subtle form of pedagogy (Freidson, 1988). The extent to which this emergent pedagogy affects student enculturation is important and provides a particular epistemological stance, in that it is a particular and unpredicted type of knowledge that students are learning which is interwoven throughout the three themes which, as O'Brien (2013) believes, are integral to workplace learning. We provide examples in the following to highlight the three interrelated themes identified in the study.

- **Work Experience** – *Students would enact behaviours of the experienced paramedics and mentors whilst working in the practice setting* (as depicted in the fieldnotes (06/04/2013)).
- **Institutionalisation** – *There was a constant mistrust and resentment by experienced paramedics and students of managers and control staff* (as depicted in the fieldnotes (20/05/2014)).
- **Professional Identity** – *Experienced paramedics (old timers) and students would display a sense of authority and power once they were wearing their green ambulance service uniform* (as depicted in the fieldnotes (02/08/2013)).

Tensions existed between what had been taught in university and what was learnt in the practice setting. This was due, in part, to the perceptions and values of stakeholders involved in the practice environment. For example, student paramedics perceptions and values emerged from the formal taught curriculum whilst in university (Donaghy, 2010). Experienced paramedic practitioners displayed a very different perception of students (Devenish, 2014), who were often depicted as 'newbies', an additional burden, who needed to be watched, thus adding to the complexity and responsibility of the paramedic's already, busy shift. There was little, if any, understanding of the student's role. Some paramedic mentors took an interest in trying to understand the students' university course to try and help support the students and sympathise with the challenges they faced in the practice setting, whilst others showed little, if any, interest in helping them. We provide a further example here, taken from the fieldnotes, to help illustrate this point.

> Whilst waiting for the student to arrive for his shift, I was speaking with Andrew (Andy), an experienced paramedic with 12 years operational experience. We were discussing university students and I quickly gained a sense that Andy was not that keen with having a student attached to him for the shift. He was derogatory about the process, stating that he was 'fed up with it, having students with me all the time, looking after them, pampering them and trying to teach them, it grinds you down, you know gets on your tits'.
>
> Taken from my fieldnotes (14/04/2014).

Boychuck Duchscher and Cowin (2004) reiterate the concept of marginalisation to help illustrate how nurses in North America became disadvantaged and discriminated against when in the clinical workplace setting, for example, by stigmatisation and labelling of newly qualified nurses in their first year by senior staff. This resulted in frequent references to the newly qualified nurses as 'new graduates, kids, young nurses, novices, newbies, as distinct from seasoned, senior, or expert nurses' (Boychuck Duchscher & Cowin, 2004: 291). Cowin and Hengstberger-Sims (2004) challenge the way the education system prepares student nurses for the workplace, offering a view that it is essentially at odds with nursing care philosophy. We looked at paramedic students in our study and how they had to learn the hidden curriculum drawn from the entrenched subculture of the workplace. We thought about the ritualistic routines of day-to-day work, since failure to understand this meant students would not be accepted by the experienced paramedics and subsequent community of practice (Lave and Wenger, 1991). We provide an example here, taken from the data, to help illustrate this.

> Whilst I was riding out with Thomas the student, and Rachel the paramedic, I was surprised to learn that two students from the previous year's university cohort had failed their practice placements. Rachel explained: 'They were nice enough kids but just didn't fit in, you know, wanted to do their own thing rather than accept the way things are done around here' (Observational fieldnotes recorded on 12/04/2013 whilst riding returning to station with Thomas and Rachel).

Some forms of knowledge are being absorbed by students during their engagement in the processes of their work experience, institutionalisation, and development of professional identity. Students began to doubt the knowledge they received at university, as anything more than an abstract concept, and were confused as to their responsibilities in their new role, which can also be seen in the work of Boychuck Duchscher (2009). These feelings and experiences served to form students' ontological position in the real world (Sharar, 2016) and how students became integral to, and formed part of, the community of experienced practitioners, similar to those which Lave and Wenger (1991: 65) illustrate in their 'work on Yucatec midwives, Vai and Gola tailors, naval quartermasters and meat cutters'.

Our findings illustrate that this matters deeply with regard to students who want to identify with the experienced paramedic community as it sees itself. The way in which the paramedics see themselves was not always the same as the professional body, regulatory authority, Health Education England, and universities may envisage. The relationship between the classroom and situated clinical practice highlighted a lack of coherence between that taught in university (McLaughlin et al., 2012) and the reality of the practice environment. Mulder et al. (2019) found a great deal of what occurs in the workplace context is not prescribed nor foreseen in curriculum documents. For example, students were taught in the university classroom how regulation, professional accountability, and formal processes govern graduate paramedic development, which includes professional standards of conduct, performance, and ethics (Health & Care Professions Council, 2016; Quality Assurance Agency, 2016) as essential attributes for graduates. The values and behaviours of graduate paramedics, whilst working alongside other healthcare professionals, such as doctors, nurses, and allied health professionals, also contribute to the essential criteria for graduate paramedics in meeting the expectations of patients, the professional body, and the UK regulator. Yet, our findings were not necessarily conducive to this notion. To shed light on this, Burford et al. (2014) imply that students develop in a vacuum of moral dilemma and professional integrity. van der Gaag and Donaghy's (2013: 8) 'analysis over an eight-year period found that the majority of complaints about registered health professionals concerned conduct, not competence'. This implies that the behaviours and experiences of paramedics may go beyond the workplace in some instances which may extend into private as well as work domains. Students became isolated, at times marginalised, and unsure once in clinical practice, as the experienced paramedics did not always display professional behaviour to one another and towards the students and other healthcare professionals. This is because some of the learning which occurs in the practice setting is about cultural norms, behaviours, and values of the practitioner which is partly due to the hidden curriculum and is recognised in several different studies, such as Lempp and Seale (2004), Kramer (1974), Metz (1981), Corman (2017), Palmer (1983), and Mannon (1992). The theory of a hidden curriculum forms part of the theorisation of this work, as we needed to understand why students have little control of their learning experience once they are enculturated into the day-to-day practices, customs, and traditions of the ambulance service workplace. Becker et al.'s (1961) work, on medical students in the USA, found the challenges, misconceptions, and relationship between the students and faculty proved difficult and unexpected, such as working extremely long hours, the volume and detail of information they were expected to absorb each day, and the poor working conditions experienced in their practical anatomy laboratory (labs), which became a form of debate amongst the students at every opportunity. This helped us to review student paramedics and the often hostile and challenging environment they become exposed to in their clinical workplace. We used Lave and Wenger's (1991) work, to help further understand what was happening here, as they liken practice learning as a way newcomer's move from being peripheral participants, working under instruction from their mentor or master as a novice, through to becoming fully legitimate participants, working as experienced autonomous practitioners (expert). We then wondered if this was an inevitable part of the enculturation process which students must go through. We therefore looked at Benner's (1984) model of learning to provide a useful reminder of how students move through the learning process from novice to expert, along with Geertz's (1973) work of how people experience life and the cultural ideologies of behaviour within organisations. We propose that it is reasonable to surmise from our findings that some student paramedics became marginalised (Boychuck Duchscher & Cowin, 2004) within the working culture of seasoned paramedic practitioners, as Lave and Wenger hypothesise that learning theories are positioned on underlying assumptions about the person, the world, and their relations, which they argue formulates social practice, which in turn generates situated activity, often treated separately from that of formal classroom education (Lave & Wenger, 1991) as opposed to that which takes place in the workplace. Our work depicts learning as a social process, occurring within the communities of the workplace. Little common ground existed between the university classroom learning and that of the workplace. Some of the taught elements of classroom education provided at university conflicted with the busy, pressured, practical workplace setting of the ambulance service as depicted in the work of McCann et al. (2013) and Corman (2017).

So far, this chapter has depicted a form of learning which student paramedics are exposed to. This learning is often covert and subtle in nature. It is a form of learning experience which is drawn from the hidden curriculum of the paramedics' working environment, as students become enculturated into a very different community. Considering the aforementioned discussions, the next section of the chapter illustrates how students form an integral part of the community of practice. The unwitting and implicit part of their learning, which many students were not consciously aware of, are unpacked and examined.

## 6.5 Communities of practice and storytelling

Students embarked on a journey whilst in the practice setting, which Lave and Wenger (1991) regard as learners going from a state of being on the peripheral of their working community, to one of full membership. This was not a conscious act; instead, it was a covert process which took place over weeks and months. Sometimes, a significant incident, such as taking charge of looking after a patient, would help build student confidence. An example of this, taken from my observational fieldnotes, illustrates this in the following.

Once again, I witnessed the eagerness of the student to please the paramedic mentor. Here Tony (student) was really getting involved in helping to treat and manage a very sick person, Jim (experienced paramedic and mentor) appeared pleased with Tony's performance and congratulated him after the incident at the hospital (Observational fieldnotes recorded on 14/11/2014 whilst ridding out with Tony and Jim).

These events were significant, increasing student confidence and promoting the legitimacy of their position within the team, although rare. The impact of this positive feedback gave students a sense of belonging as they became an integral part of the team. Students were expected to understand the various practices and roles they were to perform. Membership to these teams or communities gave students a form of identity, which Tangherlini (2000) identifies as being anti-heroes, confiding only within their own unique communities and engaging in storytelling as a predominant factor within their cultural environment, as also found in the work of Mannon (1992) and Metz (1981). We found the storytelling consisted of the paramedic's own unique working experiences, pertaining to incidents they had attended during the shift (see Chapter 5). An example from the fieldnotes is given here.

We arrived back at the ambulance station after a busy late turn shift. Jennie, the student, went straight into the watch-room. As I arrived at the watch-room, some short time afterwards, Jennie was reiterating to two other students how we had struggled to extricate a large elderly female from her flat earlier that day. There was a great deal of laughter and jovial comments and actions as Jennie gave explicit detail of the patient's poor personal hygiene and infected ulcerated legs (Observational fieldnotes recorded back on station on 19/03/2014 whilst riding out with Jennie, the student paramedic).

Whist at Giddins general hospital, I met up with several university students from various ambulances who had just handed over their patients to the Accident and Emergency (A&E) department staff. They informed me of various incidents (jobs) they had attended that day. One student expressing how he had dealt with 'time wasters' all day. I asked him what he meant by 'time wasters', he replied, 'you know the druggies and piss artists' (Observational fieldnotes recorded on 11/08/2014 whilst the crew were handing over the patient to the nursing staff at hospital).

Tangherlini (2000) found these types of conversations were often drawn out, as other crew members would interject with similar tales of their own unique stories, what Tangherlini refers to as *war stories*. We were mindful of Mannon's (1992) work and the appetite he found when the emergency medical technicians and paramedics returned to quarters (ambulance station). Here, they were able to express their feelings whilst they interacted within their unique ambulance station community. To situate this work, Corman (2017), McCann et al. (2013), Lovegrove (2013), Tangherlini (2000), Mannon (1992), Metz (1981), and Palmer (1983) found unique work-based communities formed the very fabric of the paramedics' shift. As our findings reveal these stories had a sense of companionship as various stories were discussed, whilst jovial behaviour was played out. Students became complacent in accepting the various stories and tales afforded them by the experienced paramedics and which Palmer (1983) found with rookies (new paramedics) who were initiated into the workplace by the old-timers' 'blood & guts' stories. These stories helped cement the foundations of becoming accepted into the community, as students deciphered and learned to accept these often lengthy and at times outrageous stories. Palmer (1983), Corman (2017), and

Metz (1981) also show how rookies would be drawn into storytelling as a means of acceptance into their working environment. We provide an illustration here, taken from the fieldnotes, to help highlight this.

---

I was on a night shift with Ann the student and Richard the experienced paramedic. I recall sitting in the back of the ambulance (Saloon) at 03:30 in the morning whilst Richard was recalling an incident, he had attended about 15 years ago.

Richard was explicitly and graphically, explaining to Ann, who was sitting in the ambulance cab next to Richard, about a patient who he had attended in the city and who had been struck by a train (a person being struck or fallen under a train, is commonly known to paramedics as a 'one under'). Although some 15 years previously, I remember how Richard was still able to recall all the gory graphic details of the incident (job). I looked at Ann, whilst Richard continued to explain, how he had to crawl under the train to reach the patient. Using only a touch light for visibility as he wriggled along the track under the train, before stumbling across a severed leg. He explains how there were bits of bone and body parts scattered along the track until he finally reached the main torso and part of the patient's head. Ann looked shocked but was keen to hear more, asking Richard, how they moved the body etc. (Observational fieldnotes taken whilst I was riding out with Richard, the experienced paramedic, and Ann, the student paramedic on 07/12/2014 whist travelling in the ambulance on-route back to the ambulance station).

Taken from my fieldnotes (07/12/2014).

---

The works of Moskos (2008), Corman (2017), Mannon (1992), and Palmer (1983) illustrate similar forms of storytelling, which further note the essential components of the practice setting, along with the cultural inferences which develop. They give rise to a form of community in which outsiders, such as members of the public, other healthcare workers, and even some other emergency services, form little, if any, part of, and therefore are unable to understand the uniqueness in which this community operates.

The form of storytelling revealed common values and understanding of when and who these integrate 'blood & guts' stories could be told. Students now understand the unwritten, unheard, and unspoken rules of 'engagement'.

This storytelling or folklore (Tangherlini, 2000) provides a form of behaviour, often unseen and unknown by those outside the paramedic community. In the next section, we illustrate the tensions experienced by students in the workplace, as we uncover the relationship between crew staff and managers, which are evident within our findings.

## 6.6 Tensions

Students experienced a form of tension that was, in part, due to the behaviours of experienced paramedics, which students later confirmed to me were often difficult to manage or challenge. Becker et al.'s (1961) work found tensions existed between medical students and the university faculty. The sense of community amongst medical students had become a powerful experience for students. Becker et al. (1961) found camaraderie existed amongst year groups, as opposed to those of authority within the faculty. Pratt et al. (2006) provide an alternative example, suggesting different identities exist between medical communities, for example between surgeons, anaesthetists, radiologists, and so on. This is due to their status within society, along with the presence of their learned societies, such as the British Medical Association (BMA), the Royal College of Anaesthetists, the Royal College of Radiologists, and the Royal College of Surgeons. They consider this as a central premise of the medical community. To try and make sense of this, Lipsky (2010) provides a degree of insight, suggesting the concept of street-level bureaucracy gauged his ethnographic observations of the day-to-day vicissitudes of frontline public servants, such as police officers, medical staff, housing officers, probation officers, and teachers (see Chapter 5) to help understand the wider landscape, along with the comparativeness of these workplace communities as opposed to the more elite members of society.

Having acknowledged that various forms of tension are evident in our data, we set out to show how this weaved through the narrative of the data which consisted of tensions between experienced staff, such as the old-timers, and student paramedics. We found students struggling to manage these tensions, as many experienced paramedics (old-timers) often appeared disinterested, demoralised, and demotivated, which was evident in their day-to-day work, such as taking an ambulance out of commission (not able to attend an emergency call), claiming that they had a soiled (dirty) uniform, meaning they would need to go back to the ambulance station to change, and so on. Wankhade and Mackway-Jones (2015) infer that the experienced old-timers feel the new cadre of paramedics (students) have developed at a pace which is not reflective of the realities of the road (doing the job). This tension is what Tuckman (1965) and Belbin (1981) attribute to the forming and storming processes, referring to how the construction of teams or groups are formed and emerge in particular patterns, see also Spataro (2019). Tensions can emerge as groups are formed and constructed. Further explanation is required as it impacted on student engagement in the learning process, as there was a reluctance and apparent inability by students to challenge the poor behaviour of experienced members of staff whilst in the practice setting.

This can be answered in part, as crew staff and managers left students' little opportunity to raise concerns with the higher levels of authority. The risk of being ostracised from their (student) cultural group was not an option.

Considering the aforementioned discussions, Blaber (2015) suggests that an essential premise of student development, is a safe, secure and supportive practice placement and an essential component of student learning. Jones et al. (2010) explored the emotional and mental strain that first responders became exposed to which affected the mental wellbeing of the individuals. This poses a unique and contentious issue because the learning process became stifled and entrenched within the hidden curriculum to which students were being exposed, so the student's health and wellbeing became difficult to measure (Boyle et al., 2008), as they were unable to challenge the experienced staff or gain support within the organisation. McCall et al.'s (2009) work found deficits existed in the relationship which impeded the fostering of quality clinical paramedic education in a UK ambulance service. Students were unprepared; there was little, if any, preparation to adequately communicate the learning they were about to experience in the clinical placement setting. Identification of problems early, particularly in relation to student support, is an essential element of care. McCall et al. (2009) found good supervisor/mentor relationships were key components of the students' learning, whilst Devenish (2014) found some socialisation of student paramedics occurred in the university setting prior to their clinical practice placements. He refers to the work of Cant and Higgs (1999) in recognising the juxtaposition of formal textbook descriptions of the paramedic curriculum, as opposed to that portrayed in practice. Cant and Higgs (1999: 49) suggest this is 'fraught with conflicts and confusions for students to grapple with'. The following example illustrates where a student learned that academic study was sometimes frowned upon in the practice setting.

---

Whilst sitting in the ambulance outside the hospital, (Jim) the student, started to read a paramedic journal. Whilst we were discussing several articles in the journal, I asked him if he reads this journal back at the ambulance station in the watch-room. Jim replied, 'no way, I normally have something with me to read relating to the job (paramedic profession) but I only get that out of my bag once I have established who I am working with and no way would I read it on station, I get enough grief as it is, without encouraging it' (Observational fieldnotes taken whilst I was riding out on an ambulance with Jim, the student paramedic, these notes were recorded as we were at the hospital and the paramedic had gone off to the canteen (22/09/2015).

Taken from my fieldnotes (22/09/2015).

The aforementioned example illustrates a form of conflict this student experienced between university and work experience. It provides an outline of what really happens in practice and it gets to the heart of how sharply the cultural inclinations of the student clashed with the guys on the road, often with consequent negative implications for pedagogy and best practice. Students' learning became influenced by a deep-rooted sense of negativity, which was frequently displayed by the more experienced paramedics. Devenish (2014) found conflicts existed between the older traditionally trained workforce and the younger university workforce. The following example provides insight into the traditional culture experienced by the students in our study.

> Although (Roy) is a newly qualified paramedic (NQP), he is very territorial and overrides students or constantly appears to question the decisions with patients whilst the student is questioning the patient at the time. Rebecca, the student, appeared to stop talking, not challenging Roy, but rather accepts his authority as a NQP and just works under his instructions. This did not appear to be mentorship, but a form of power (Observational fieldnotes recorded on the 12/04/2013 whilst I was riding out with the crew).

The aforementioned example illustrates a common thread which weaved throughout the data. It is significant, because the newly qualified paramedics (NQPs) themselves were likely to be paramedic graduates, yet behaved in ways that could be more associated with the old-timers. This observation is examined further in the next section of this chapter as the notion of professional identity is explored.

## 6.7 Professional identity or blue-collar workers

Professional identity emerged out of the data as a discrete yet powerful theme and one which needs further understanding to help position this theme within the context of the subculture. However, Pillen et al. (2013) imply the concept of professionalism, along with professional identity, is varied and difficult to define. Freidson (2004) argues that professionalism consists of knowledge that is esoteric not because it is mysterious, but because it is unique, and takes time and effort to acquire. We looked at Goltz and Smith (2014) to provide a useful understanding of professional identity as '[a] form of social identification that individuals have within, and of, a profession, such as medicine, law, nursing etc'. They go on to suggest:

> The degree in which individuals define themselves as members of a profession, and thereon their professional identity, consists of the

individual's alignment of various roles, responsibilities, values and ethical standards which are consistent with practices accepted by the specific profession.

(Goltz & Smith, 2014: 785–789)

Pratt et al. (2006) found that identity construction was triggered by work-identity integrity violations. Suggesting that, a mismatch existed between what physicians did and who they were. These violations were resolved through identity customisation processes as part of an interrelated identity and work learning cycles.

Our findings illustrate professional identity is an inherent component of the data. Issues such as the paramedics' distinctive, idiosyncratic, green uniforms, as Tangherlini (2000) and Lovegrove (2013) imply, influence the importance that the paramedic uniforms provide, both for the public and paramedics themselves. The paramedics' identity became an integral part of the behaviours and customs which reinforced the social context in which this work is positioned (see Chapter 5). The green paramedic uniform acted as a conduit which illustrated a sense of authority, identity, and professional status (Reynolds, 2007). Displayed throughout the data collection, this formed a visual symbol of authority and expertise (Lazarsfeld-Jensen, 2014). This identity was relevant, both internally, within the organisational rank structure of the ambulance service, and externally by the immediately recognisable uniform of paramedics.

We would argue, however, that crews lacked a sense of autonomy, restricted by formal processes and controls. McCann et al. (2013) found that crews are tethered and leashed and have little autonomy, as crews become governed and therefore dependent upon delivery of various targets, deadlines, and schedules. For example, whilst I was riding out collecting data, I saw how every aspect of our working day was monitored, such as the time it took to attend a call, the time spent at the scene of a call, the time taken to drive to hospital, and, more importantly, downtime (time not available to attend calls), whilst at the hospital. These were all electronically monitored and recorded by the mobile data tracking (MDT) system. This illustrates how paramedic crews are controlled, monitored, and restricted in their day-to-day working practices, which we further argue are not necessarily conducive to autonomy. McCann et al. (2013), along with Wankhade and Mackway-Jones (2015), found paramedic crews and students are governed by these electronic tags, albeit from the mobile data terminal in the ambulance, the phone and computer in station, the radio from ambulance control, which is positioned in the ambulance cab, and the portable radio always carried by the paramedic crews. Furthermore, crew members attending the bathroom were still subject to receiving an emergency call, as identified by McCann et al. (2013). Hafler et al. (2011) suggest these practices and processes are not helpful when decoding the learning environment, whilst Cribb (2008) suggests that these types of practice form part of organisational control. Corman (2017) and McCann et al. (2013) found paramedics personally interpret these restrictions and then construct their own occupational professional identity, like those which Lipsky (2010) identifies, just as paramedics in our study would turn their portable radio off when using the bathroom in defiance to alleviate this pressure. This does not convey a sense of professionalism, although our findings reveal both students and experienced paramedics had a strong sense of professional identity which was explicit and striking, and there was a sense of power, authority, status, purpose, and community. Examples of these are provided in the following, taken from the fieldnotes.

Student paramedics and experienced paramedics would often act like police officers to gain control of situations, such as domestic disputes which had resulted in an injury to one of the parties (Observational fieldnotes recorded on 11/05/2015 whilst I was riding out with the crew).

Members of the public appeared to expect and accept some kind of order to be restored, to an often-chaotic scene, as we (ambulance crew) arrived at the emergency call (Observational fieldnotes recorded on 02/03/2014 whilst I was riding out with the crew).

Sarros et al. (2002) liken this style of control illustrated earlier to a bureaucratic, quasi-military type organisation. O'Meara (2009) provides deeper understanding of paramedic identity, whilst Reynolds (2004) helps illustrate this phenomenon. O'Meara suggests registration and regulation are components of professional identity, both of which are synonymous with the UK paramedics, whilst Donaghy (2012) believes registration and regulation are essential components in enhancing the professionalisation of paramedics to the next level. Lipsky (2010) refers to the realities of street-level practice, suggesting the work becomes far removed from abstract ideologies, such as professionalisation, as also seen in the work of Burford (2012). This is not the professional identity seen by those who promote the development of the profession, such as the College of Paramedics (COP), Health Education England (HEE), Council of Deans of Health (COD), the Health and Care Professions Council (HCPC), and the Association of Ambulance Chief Executives (AACE). Instead, these are aspects of professional identity that grow out of the realities of the working practices, reiterating the hidden curriculum. O'Meara (2009) suggests that:

The evolving professionalism of paramedics needs to be confirmed through professional behaviours that incorporate adherence to professional codes of conduct, reflective practice and commitment to continuing professional development.

(O'Meara, 2009: 2)

Reynolds' (2004) review of professional development of paramedics in Australia suggests progress has been slow. The sense of what is understood by professionalisation, as evidenced in the paramedics' workplace, appeared somewhat limited. Accordingly, we found students' observations of practice led to a form of confusion regarding the expectations of professionalism (Zubin et al., 2005), as students sometimes encountered disruption and conflict, as a result of the use of varying forms of racism, sexism, and bullying whilst on the road (see Chapter 5). Students were expected to participate in the traditional working practices and processes inherent within the workplace setting, and these sometimes included meal break avoidance, off jobs (finishing their shifts on time), writing graffiti on the walls of ambulance stations, bullying, and vehicle sabotage (cutting and exposing electrical wires). We found cultural integration into the paramedics' community of practice (Lave & Wenger, 1991) was often associated with bullying and stereotyping, as documented in the findings. Students became aware of the possible consequences of non-conformity, that is they became rejected, abandoned, and, according to Boychuck Duchscher (2009), marginalised. They often acted as larger-than-life characters, super-heroes, and authoritative in their distinctive green uniforms (Lovegrove, 2013; Tangherlini, 2000) to make an impression as they grappled with their perceived professional identity. They formulated cynical views and assumptions about patients, which they would often claim to be examples of dark humour (see Chapter 5). However, we argue this did not correspond to dark humour, but a reflection of the intricacies and nuances of observed behaviour that weaved through the students' day-to-day practices. This formed part of the subculture which existed. These are all examples of the disparity between the formal university classroom learning and that of the practice setting, which operates as a hidden curriculum, unplanned and unintended by policy makers and university programmes.

Selected theoretical models of enculturation have been discussed in this chapter. These models rely on the work of Lave and Wenger's (1991) communities of practice, Becker et al.'s (1961) study of medical students, and Schein's (1985) model of organisational culture. In formulating these theoretical concepts, we were reminded of the work of many other authors who have contributed to this section of work. Drawing on the findings, we have illustrated the many challenges and demands placed upon the student. Our findings also reveal this workplace culture is often unchallenged and uncritically accepted. The following section of this chapter sets out the implications for practice on student enculturation.

## 6.8 Implications for practice

The implications for practice, stemming from the findings, serve to strengthen the need for further research in this area. For any significant change to occur within the profession, the work experiences and professional identity, along with the stringent structurally confined organisation, need to be addressed. Our findings reveal that accumulatively this can inhibit and detract from any significant change at all levels (Givati et al., 2018), to include both the micro (individual) level and the macro (organisational, institutional, and professional) level. In this section, we address the implications for practice before offering suggestions for change in the next chapter (Chapter 7) and suggest potential solutions in tackling the subculture and hidden curriculum depicted within the NHS ambulance service trust.

This work lays claim that learning styles are contextually linked to the cultural setting. For example, Lave and Wenger (1991) express how learners or new trainees contextualise their learning experiences to their situational participation, such as those of their experienced paramedic colleagues and mentors. This raises a key question arising from the study, which is what is taught in the university classroom is not necessarily sufficient to equip students for the culturally based practices embedded within the ambulance and paramedic working environment. The university curriculum focuses on the award of a degree (Ball, 2005). This is not always reflective or necessarily aligned to current trends and working practices carried out in the workplace, which Hafferty (1998) and O'Donnell (2014) suggest. In addressing these issues, a structurally work-based approach is required to accurately reflect the realities of the practice setting, without diluting the key components of knowledge, skills, and practice, required to produce paramedic practitioners, who are fit for purpose, fit for the award of degree, and fit for practice. Nevertheless, any kind of meaningful and tangible development or adjustment to the paramedic programme would require a multi-faceted approach, involving the inclusion of the professional body, ambulance managers, educationalists, academic tutors (institutionalisation), experienced paramedics, paramedic mentors, paramedic students, service users, and trade unionists (professional identity) in the course design, development, and delivery of service. A multi-faceted partnership which draws together knowledge, experience, standards, and governance, to produce a curriculum, suitable and workable, for both the academic components of paramedic professional practice, together with the practicalities and 'real-life' issues which can taint and distort that found in the working environment of clinical practice. It could be argued that the requirements for this are already in all the relevant standards. However, it is unclear whether important voices or perspectives are lost in the process of involving and engaging these different groups.

## 6.9 Conclusion

To help contextualise how and why these findings became so relevant to this piece of work, we have illustrated how the notion of enculturation and the subsequent hidden curriculum became embedded within work cultures (Guufberg et al., 2010) in similar organisations, to that of the ambulance service, such as Sarros et al.'s (2002) work with the fire service in the USA and Lipsky's (2010) work with the American police officers. We provide an ethnographic account of how we found students in our study became shaped and conditioned into a hidden curriculum. We explored how this hidden curriculum was not that expected or planned within the wider aspects of paramedic development, situated in university education, rather a hidden curriculum drawn from the subculture which revealed a form of pedagogy unknown to, and unseen by, students, as also supported by the work of Mulder et al. (2019), O'Donnell (2014), and Hafferty and Franks (1994). Furthermore, the work addresses the fragmentation of communities of practice which became evident. Dewey (1963) offers a degree of insight by suggesting that competencies, as a system of knowledge, skills, and attitudes, may not necessarily be covered in the classroom setting. Lave (2010) suggests that learning does not begin with goals and objectives and that it begins with experience and reflection of the experience, suggesting that learning is situated and therefore is influenced and informed by the practice environment. Dreyfus (2001) claims that students firstly learn the rules of the discipline (novice), before applying the rules in certain context (advanced beginner) and then accepting the responsibility (competent) of their practice, also see Benner's (1984) model of *novice to expert*.

We have illustrated how the data drawn out of the ethnography interacts with the empirical evidence-based and pre-existing concepts such as communities of practice, workplace culture, and institutionalisation. The chapter has extracted, reviewed, critiqued, and analysed key elements of the findings within the study, and selected theoretical models of enculturation have been discussed.

The next chapter looks at the future directions and recommendations for policy and practice, along with the student assessment process, strengths and limitations of the study, and insider/outsider roles, before summarising and drawing this work to a conclusion.

## References

Andarvazh, R. M., Afshar, L. & Yazdani, S. (2017) 'Hidden curriculum: An analytical definition', *Journal of Medical Education*, 16(4), pp. 198–207.

Ball, L. (2005) 'Setting the science for the paramedic in primary care', *Emergency Medical Journal*, pp. 896–900.

Bain, L. L. (1985) 'The hidden curriculum re-examined', *Quest*, 37(2), pp. 145–153.

Becker, H., Geer, B., Hughes, C. E. & Strauss, L. A. (1961) *Boys in White*. New Brunswick, NJ: Transaction Books.

Belbin., M. (1981) *Management Teams: Why They Succeed or Fail*. London: Honeymoon.

Benner, P. (1984) *From Novice to Expert: Excellence and Power in Clinical Nursing Practice*. English – 1 January 1984. London/Sydney/Toronto/Mexico/New Delhi/Toxio/Singapore/Rio de Janeiro: Prentice Hall.

Billett, S. (2002) 'Workplace pedagogic practices: Co–participation and learning', *British Journal of Educational Studies*, 50(4), pp. 457–481.

Blaber, A. (2015) *The Student Paramedic Survival Guide: Journey from Student to Paramedic*, 2015 ed. New York: McGraw-Hill Education.

Boychuck Duchscher, J. E. (2009) 'Transition shock: The initial stage of role adaptation for newly graduated registered nurses', *Journal of Advanced Nursing*, 65(5), pp. 1103–1113.

Boychuck Duchscher, J. E. & Cowin, S. L. (2004) 'The experience of marginalisation in new nursing graduates', *Nursing Outlook*, 52, pp. 289–296.

Boyle, J. M., William, B., Cooper, J., Adams, B. & Alford, K. (2008) 'Ambulance clinical placements: A pilot study of student' experience', *British Medical Education*, 8, p. 19. https://doi.org/10.1186/1472-6920-8-19

Brewer, J. D. (1991) *Inside the RUC*. Oxford: Oxford University Press.

Brewer, J. D. (2000) *Ethnography: Understanding Social Research*. Berkshire/New York: Open University Press.

Brown, D. (2002) 'The role of work and cultural values in occupational choice, satisfaction, and success: A theoretical statement', *Journal of Counselling & Development*, 80(1), pp. 48–56.

Burford, B. (2012) 'Group processes in medical education: Learning from social identity theory', *Medical Education*, 46(2), pp. 143–152.

Burford, B., Morrow, G., Rothwell, C., Carter, M. & Illing, J. (2014) 'Group processes in medical education: Learning from social identity theory', *Medical Education*, 48(4), pp. 361–375.

Burns, R. J. (2002) 'Education and social change: A proactive or reactive role'? *International Review of Education*, 48(1), pp. 21–45.

Campbell, D., Shepherd, I., McGrail, M., Kassell, L., Connolly, M., Williams, B. & Nestel, D. (2015) 'Procedural skills practice and training needs of doctors, nurses, midwives and paramedics in rural Victoria', *Advances in Medical Education and Practice*, 19(6), pp. 183–194.

Cant, R. & Higgs, J. (1999) 'Professional socialisation in educating beginning practitioners', in J. Higgs & H. Edwards (Eds.), *Educating Beginning Practitioners: Challenges for Health Professional Education* (pp. 46–51). Oxford: Butterworth-Heinemann.

Corman, K. M. (2016) 'Street medicine – Assessment work strategies of paramedics on the front lines of emergency health services', *Journal of Contemporary Ethnography*, 46(5), pp. 600–623.

Corman, K. M. (2017) *Paramedics On and Off the Streets-Emergency Medical Services in the Age of Technological Governance*. Toronto/Buffalo/London: University of Toronto Press.

Cowin, L. S. & Hengstberger-Sims, C. (2004) 'New graduate nurse self-concept and retention: A longitudinal survey', *International Journal of Nursing Studies* 43, 59–70.

Crawford, J. & Lok, P. (1999) 'The relationship between commitment and organizational culture, subculture, leadership style and job satisfaction in organizational change and development', *Leadership & Organization Development Journal*, 20(7), pp. 365–373.

Cribb, A. (2008) *Whose Responsibility? Changing Teacher Professionalism: International Trends, Challenges and Ways Forward*. London: Routledge, p. 31.

Devenish, A. S. (2014) 'Experiences in becoming a paramedic: A qualitative study examining the university qualified paramedics', *Creative Education*, 7(6), pp. 786–801.

Dewey, J. (1963) *Experience and Education*. First publ. New York, NY: Collier Books.

Donaghy, J. (2010) 'Equipping the student for the workplace changes in paramedic education', *Journal of Paramedic Practice*, 2(11), pp. 524–528.

Donaghy, J. (2012) *Specialist Development Roles for the Paramedic. Foundations for Paramedic Practice: A Theoretical Perspective*, 2nd ed. New York: Mc Graw Hill.

Dreyfus, H. (2001) *On the Internet*. London, England: Routledge Press.

Freidson, E. (1988) *A Study of the Sociology of Applied Knowledge*, 2nd ed. Chicago/ London: University of Chicago Press.

Freidson, E. (2004) *Professionalism, the Third Logic*, 2nd ed. Cambridge/Malden: Policy Press.

Freire, P. (1985) *The Politics of Education: Culture Power and Liberation*. London: McMillan.

Geertz, C. (1973) *The Interpretation of Cultures*. New York, NY: Basic Books.

Giroux, A. H. & Penna, N. A. (2012) 'Social education in the classroom: The dynamics of the hidden curriculum', *Theory & Research in Social Education*, 7(1), pp. 21–42.

Givati, A., Markham, C. & Street, K. (2018) 'The bargaining of professionalism in emergency care practice: NHS paramedics and higher education', *Advances in Health Science Education*, 23, p. 353.

Goltz, H. H. & Smith, M. L. (2014) 'Forming and developing your professional identity: Easy as PI', *Health Promotion Practice*, 15(6), pp. 785–789.

Guufberg, H. H., Batalden, M., Sanda, R. & Bell, S. K. (2010) 'The hidden curriculum, what can we learn from third-year medical student narrative reflections?', *Academic Medicine*, 85, pp. 1709–1716.

Hafferty, F. W. (1998) 'Beyond curriculum reform: Confronting medicine's hidden curriculum', *Academic Medicine*, 73(4), pp. 403–407.

Hafferty, F. W. & Franks, R. (1994) 'The hidden curriculum, ethics teaching and the structure of medical education', *Academic Medicine*, 69, pp. 861–871.

Hafferty, F. W. & O'Donnell, J. F. (2014) *The Hidden in Curriculum in Health Professional Education*, 1st ed. Hanover, New Hampshire: Dartmouth College Press.

Hafler, P. J., Ownby, R. A., Thompson, M. B., Fasser, E. C., Grigsby, K. Haidet, P. Kahn, J. M. & Hafferty, W. F. (2011) 'Decoding the learning environment of medical: A hidden curriculum perspective for faculty development', *Academic Medicine*, 86(4), pp. 440–444.

Health and Care Professions Council (HCPC). (2016) *Health Care Professions Council – Social Work*. http://www.hcpc-uk.org/aboutregistration/professions/ index.asp?id=18#profDetails (Accessed 2nd February 2016).

Henderson, R. (2011) 'Classroom pedagogies, digital literacies and the home-school digital divide', *International Journal of Pedagogies and Learning*, 6(2), pp. 152–161.

Jackson, P. W. (1968) *Life in Classrooms*. New York, NY: Holt, Reinhart & Winston.

Jones, A., Slater, J. & Griffiths, P. (2010) 'The first year experiences of paramedic students in higher education: A mixed evaluation', in *Health Science and Practice*. Swansea: London Higher Education Academy, p. 37. https://cronfa.swan.ac.uk/ Record/cronfa24957

Kelly, A. V. (2006) *The Curriculum Theory and Practice*, 5th ed. London/Thousand Oaks/New Delhi: SAGE Publishing.

Kramer, M. (1974) *Reality Shock: Why Nurses Leave Nursing*. St Louis: C.V. Mosby Company.

Lave, J. (2010) 'Teaching, as learning, in Practice', *Journal of Mind, Culture and Activity*, 3(3).

Lave, J. & Wenger, E. (1991) *Situated Learning: Legitimate Peripheral Participation*. Cambridge/New York/Melbourne/Madrid/Cape Town: Cambridge University Press.

Lazarsfeld-Jensen, A. (2014) 'Telling stories out of school: Experiencing the paramedic's oral traditions and role dissonance', *Nurse Education in Practice*, 14(6), pp. 734–739.

Lempp, H. & Seale, C. (2004) 'The hidden curriculum in undergraduate medical education: Qualitative study of medical students' perceptions of teaching', *British Medical Journal*, 329 (2 October). bmj.com

Lipsky, M. (2010) *Street-Level Bureaucracy Dilemmas of the Individual in Public Services*. New York: Russel Sage Foundation.

Lord, B. (2009) 'Paramedic assessment of pain in the cognitively impaired adult patient', *BMC Emergency Medicine*, 9(1), pp. 1–9.

Lovegrove, M. & Davis, J. (2013) *Paramedic Evidence Based Education Project (PEEP): Maximising Paramedic' Contribution to the Delivery of High Quality and Cost-Effective Patient Care*. Buckinghamshire: Bucks.

Mannon, M. J. (1992) *Emergency Encounters – EMTs and Their Work*. Boston, MA: Jones and Bartlett.

Martin, J. & Siehl, C. (1983) 'Organizational culture and counterculture: An uneasy symbiosis', *Organizational Dynamics*, 12(2), pp. 52–64.

McCall, L., Wray, N. & Lord, B. (2009) 'Factors affecting the education of pre-employment paramedic students during the clinical practicum', *Journal of Emergency Primary Health Care*, 7(4).

McCann, L., Granter, E., Hyde, P. & Hassard, J. (2013) 'Still blue-collar after all these years? An ethnography of the professionalisation of emergency work', *Journal of Management Studies*, 50(5), pp. 750–774.

McLaughlin, H., Ugreen, C. & Blackstone, A. (2012) 'Sexual harassment, workplace, authority, and the paradox of power', *American Sociological*, 77(40), pp. 625–647.

Metz, L. D. (1981) *Running Hot-Structure and Stress in Ambulance Work*, 1st ed. Edited by L. D. Metz. Cambridge, MA: Abt Books.

Moore, P. (2000) 'Research, reality and "hanging around"', *Sociology Review*, 10(3), pp. 8–13.

Moskos, P. C. (2008) *Cop in the Hood: My Year Policing Baltimore's Eastern District*. Princeton/Oxford: Princeton University Press.

Mulder, H., ter Braak, E., Chen, C. H. & ten Cate, O. (2019) 'Addressing the hidden curriculum in the clinical workplace: A practical tool for trainees and faculty Addressing the hidden curriculum in the clinical workplace: A practical tool for trainees and faculty', *Medical Teacher*, 41(1), pp. 36–43. https://doi.org/10.1080/0 142159X.2018.1436760

O'Brien, S. (2013) 'The borrowers: Researching the cognitive aspects of translation target', *International Journal of Translation Studies*, 25(1), pp. 5–17.

O'Donnell, J. F. (2014) 'Introduction: The hidden curriculum–A focus on learning and closing the gap', in Hafferty, F. W., & O'Donnell, J. F. (Eds.), *The Hidden Curriculum in Health Professional Education*. 1st ed. Hanover, NH: Dartmouth College Press, pp. 1–20.

O'Meara, P. (2009) 'Professional and community expectations of rural ambulance services in Australia, pp2', *The Australian Journal of Paramedicine*, 1(3–4), pp. 1–7.

Palmer, E. (1983) "Trauma Junkie" and street work: Occupational behaviour of paramedics and emergency medical technicians', *Journal of Contemporary Ethnography, Urban Life*, (2), pp. 162–183.

Pillen, M., Beijaard, D. & Brok, P. D. (2013) 'Tensions in beginning teachers' professional identity development, accompanying feelings and coping strategies', *European Journal of Teacher Education*, 36(3), pp. 240–260.

Pratt, M. G., Rockmann, K. W. & Kaufmann, J. B. (2006) 'Constructing professional identity: The role of work and identity learning cycles in the customization of identity among medical residents', *Academy of Management Journal*, 49(2), pp. 235–262.

Quality Assurance Agency Benchmark Statement-Paramedic. (2016) https://dera.ioe.ac.uk/27035/1/SBS-Paramedics-16.pdf

Rankin, J. M. & Campbell, M. L. (2006) *Managing to Nurse: Inside Canada's Health Care Reform*. Toronto/Buffalo/London: University of Toronto Press.

Reynolds, J. (2007) 'Discourse of inter-professionalism', *The British Journal of Social Work*, 37(3), pp. 441–457.

Reynolds, L. (2004) 'Is prehospital care really a profession', *Journal of Emergency Primary Health Care*, 2(1–2), pp. 1–6.

Sackman, S. (1991) *Cultural Knowledge in Organizations: Exploring the Collective Mind*. London: SAGE Publishing.

Sarros, J. C., Tanewski, G. A., Winter, R. P., Santora, J. C. & Densten, I. L. (2002) 'Work alienation and organisational leadership', *British Journal of Management*, 13(4), pp. 285–304.

Schein, H. E. (1985) *Organisational Culture and Leadership*, 2nd ed. San Francisco, CA: Jossey-Bay.

Sharar, B. (2016) *Emergent Pedagogy in England. A Critical Realist Study of Structure-Agency Interactions in Higher Education*. London/New York: Routledge.

Spataro, J. (2019) *5 Attributes of Successful Teams*. https://www.microsoft.com/en-us/microsoft-365/blog/2019/11/19/5-attributes-successful-teams/

Tangherlini, R. T. (2000) 'Heroes and lies: Storytelling tactics among paramedics', *The Folklore Society, Routledge Journals*, 111(1), pp. 43–66.

Thornton, R. & Nardi, M. (1975) 'The dynamics of role acquisition', *The American Journal of Sociology*, 80(4), pp. 870–885.

Trice, H. M. & Beyer, J. M. (1993) *The Cultures of Work Organizations*. Englewood Cliffs, NJ: Prentice-Hall, Inc.

Tuckman, B. W. (1965) 'Developmental sequence in small groups', *Psychological Bulletin*, 63, 384–399.

van der Gaag, A. & Donaghy, J. (2013) 'Paramedics and professionalism: Looking back and looking forwards', *Journal of Paramedic Practice*. Mark Allen Group, 5(1), pp. 8–10.

van Maanen, J. (2011) *Tales of the Field: On Writing Ethnography*, 2nd ed. Chicago/London: The University of Chicago.

Wankhade, P. & Mackway-Jones, K. (2015) *Understanding the Management of Ambulance Services Ambulance Services: Leadership and Management Perspectives*. Cham/Heidelberg/New York/Dordrecht/London: Springer.

Wenger, E. (1998) *Communities of Practice Learning, Meaning and Identity*. Cambridge/New York/Melbourne/Madrid/Cape Town: Cambridge University Press.

Whitehead, J. (2001) 'Newly qualified staff nurses' perceptions of the role transition', *Nurse Education Today*, 10, pp. 330–339.

Zubin, A., Simpson, S. & Reynen, E. (2005) 'The fault lies not in our students, but in ourselves': Academic honesty and moral development in health professions education – Results of a pilot study in Canadian pharmacy', *Journal of Teaching in Higher Education*, 10(2), pp. 143–156.

# 7 Reflections and recommendations

## 7.1 Introduction

In this chapter, we summarise the findings and illustrate how the student assessment processes are carried out, both in university and the clinical workplace. We illustrate how the insider/outsider research perspectives impacted and informed the research, before reflecting on the study. We then offer some thoughts on the strengths and limitations of the study before suggesting some potential future research for paramedic education, offering recommendations for policy and practice, prior to concluding this book.

This research is significant because it has created new knowledge about the enculturation of university student paramedics and experienced paramedics. To date, few studies have explored this topic thoroughly drawing on an ethnographic position, from university through to the impact of work-based placements. Whilst the theories of enculturation within healthcare are not new, this work generates a theoretical model of the UK student paramedic enculturation through the ethnographic perspective of an experienced paramedic practitioner and academic, reflecting a paramedic paradigm.

Unravelling the student paramedic perspectives using observational fieldnotes, interviews, and reports, this work has captured their unique and often challenging practice experiences, which O'Reilly (2009) suggests is one of the advantages of ethnographic study. Their behaviours, situations, attitudes, and voice became key to the research as we interpreted and analysed the findings. The relationship between their practice experiences and their university experiences became evident (McCann et al., 2013; Wankhade & Mackway-Jones, 2015), as the subculture emerged (Hafferty & O'Donnell, 2014) through the research process to reveal a very different curriculum to that which students had been taught at university.

## 7.2 Summary of findings

The student paramedics' experiences of university contrasted with that of their workplace practice. This highlighted a void between the elements

DOI: 10.4324/9781032721408-7

formally taught in university and those experienced and embraced by students in the workplace, along with behaviours and attitudes. Often conflicting sets of professional values and clinical practice became evident, as students worked alongside more senior paramedic mentors and experienced staff. The differences between the formal (university) and informal workplace (hidden) curriculum were evident, as one type of pedagogy occurred in the university classroom and the other on the job dealing with patients in real-life situations of ill health, injury, mental health crises, and so on.

Our findings are supported by Devenish's (2014) work on socialisation, along with Kramer's (1974) work on newly graduated nurses, which found similar issues and concerns. For example, some experienced paramedics did not recognise students as novice practitioners were in need of further training or support, because some experienced paramedics were set in their traditional ways and working practices. Lave and Wenger (1991) suggest that this forms part of the continuum of the students' community of practice, and this is the way in which social structures are formed giving rise to socio-cognitive activities we normally view as purely cognitive.

Cognition is situated within the social structures around us, suggesting that the social structure shapes and informs our knowledge. The consideration of learning as a process of becoming a member of a sustained community of practice aligns with our findings, since the students in the research were unable to challenge the recognised established ways and customs engrained within the workplace and paramedic subculture. Shortcomings in the teaching and learning environment of the practice setting, along with the application of pedagogy in clinical practice, led some students to question the value of the workplace experience. Students reported how the practice experience offered limited value to their theoretical knowledge as they felt unable to display their newly taught knowledge and skills in the clinical practice setting. At times, their practice placement experiences were a painful and challenging process which they felt they had to accept or risk hostility from the experienced paramedics, which Boychuck Duchscher's (2009) study on newly graduated nurses describes as marginalisation. Considering these discussions, it is of concern to learn that a recent media report highlights 'thirteen counts of sexual misconduct have been reported to the police at one NHS ambulance service trust where bullying was 'normalised' which it is alleged by paramedics and other employees of the ambulance service' (Look East, 2020). We were subsequently reminded of the students in our study, who confessed that the desire to succeed and become registered paramedics constrained them to adapt to the contradictions and difficulties they experienced in the workplace. An example of the extreme conditions of practice experienced by one student in the study is illustrated in the following.

I was riding out with Susan, a third-year student paramedic. I was talk-ing with Susan alone in the ambulance cab whilst we were at Sunnymead hospital. We were discussing the university degree programme and prac-tice experience when suddenly and unexpectedly, Susan became tearful, and upset. Once Susan had settled down, I asked her 'what was wrong', and why she was so upset. I was shocked and amazed at her response, which highlighted a catalogue of sexual innuendos. Such as, forms of bullying and at times allegations of inappropriate touching throughout her three years practice placements. I was clearly in a difficult position as these events should have been reported and investigated at the time. However, Susan was adamant that she shared this information with me in confidence, as someone who she could trust. Her reasoning was this, she explains: 'John, (researcher) I only have a few weeks left on place-ment then my three years are completed and I will finally be able to reg-ister as a paramedic and go and work elsewhere, away from this awful organisation'. I was stunned at such a claim! (Observational fieldnotes recorded on 17/06/2014 whilst in the ambulance at the hospital).

It remains to be seen how students, once they become qualified paramed-ics, will apply their learning in the clinical placement setting, as students have been exposed to various forms of poor practice and learned some bad habits, although Reynolds (2004) suggests that they will not necessarily entirely jet-tison the knowledge, values, and ethical principles that they have been taught at university when they become newly qualified paramedics (NQPs). We were mindful of this and take comfort from the possibility, although there is a realistic prospect that students, once they become NQPs, may become con-ditioned into the traditional ways of working, as Devenish's (2014) work implies. Therefore, the traditional workplace culture depicted in the find-ings would not become challenged, denounced, altered, or fully addressed, as NQPs (ex-students) appear to take on the traditional, taken-for-granted cus-toms and practices of the experienced paramedics (old-timers). Metz's (1981) ethnography of paramedics and emergency medical technicians (EMTs) in the USA found little evidence to support the fact that new recruits changed or influenced the already established ways of working. This also matches the findings of Reynolds (2004) and McCann et al. (2013) who found the clini-cal workplace environment has a defined and lasting impact on students and their relationship with aspects of paramedic pedagogy.

In the previous section, we have summarised the experiences of students in the workplace; this is important as these lie at the foundation of our work. To understand how students are assessed and deemed to be successfully quali-fied paramedics, despite their problematic and conflictual workplace training experience, will add further clarity and objectivity to our research. Therefore, we have dedicated the next section to illustrate the assessment structure, both in terms of the clinical workplace and the university. This provides a contextualisation of the two assessment processes, which we believe further helps understand how students are expected to meet the standards required by the HCPC.

## 7.3 Assessment processes

At university, the students' knowledge and skills are assessed throughout the course by several methods, which include ongoing assessment of the students' clinical placement experiences by a continuous record of ongoing progress, along with their academic work. This section of the chapter illustrates the two processes, workplace, and university, whilst highlighting some of the challenges these processes present.

In the clinical workplace setting, students are provided with an individual Practice Assessment Document (PAD). This is a record of the skills and competencies which students are expected to achieve throughout their time in the clinical setting. These competencies are divided into year groups, such as year one, year two, and year three. Year one consists of students having to achieve a set of basic clinical competencies, such as scene safety, communication skills, the use of basic ambulance aid equipment, and basic patient assessment. This is followed in year two and three by the need for students to demonstrate a higher level of knowledge and competency in advanced clinical skills, such as advanced patient assessment and management (treatment), advanced clinical interventions, for example, the administration of intravenous fluids (IV), and drug calculations. There is an expectation and requirement that these competencies be assessed by a trained and qualified paramedic practice placement educator (PPED) or paramedic mentor/supervisor, although I found many incidences whereby students had difficulty obtaining ratification of these competencies due to the low number of appropriately trained and qualified PPEDs, mentors, or supervisors. This is an important limitation of the practice assessment process, as other 'experienced' paramedics, who were not necessarily trained mentors, supervisors, or PPEDs, would often sign the students' PADs in the absence of their named person. This undermines the fundamental principle of the practice placement document in ensuring that the defined and agreed standards and competencies are met. It also renders the workplace assessment process highly problematic in terms of meeting both academic and professional standards, as well as the national quality assurance agency (QAA) standards.

Students returning to university are also assessed through several different methods, for example formal written examinations in topics such as pharmacology and pathophysiology. Poster presentations and verbal presentations are used for topics such as reflective practice and communication skills, whilst written assignments are used for topics such as anatomy and physiology (A&P), leadership and management, crew-resource management, and professionalisation. In addition, practical assessments, known as OSCEs (objective structured clinical examinations), are undertaken for the assessment of practical skills, such as patient assessment, the use of ambulance equipment, and clinical interventions, for example inserting a needle and administering appropriate drugs or placing a plastic tube into the patient's airway (trachea). These combined assessment processes are designed to contextualise the learning taught in the university, which replicates that of the workplace.

The validation processes undertaken by the university's internal academic validation panel, along with the HCPC's external approval panel, form part of the integrity and validation of the approval processes of the programme. These processes are designed to ensure both validity and rigour of assessments are adhered to. However, questions are raised whether this is consistent throughout the students' clinical workplace, as we found worrying examples of poor practice which was evident on several occasions whilst collecting the observational fieldnotes. For example, I found paramedics with no formal mentorship training or qualifications 'signing off' students' work, assessing their clinical skills, and grading their patient assessment in the workplace. An example of this taken from the fieldnotes helps to illustrate these practices.

> Whilst I was riding out with Amy the student paramedic, she was talking with Tony, the paramedic about her PAD document and getting it signed off by a mentor. Clearly Amy was keen to get her PAD signed, and up to date. Without hesitation, Tony took her PAD and asked Amy where she needs it signed, stating 'I will sign this for you love, you are a nice kid and I don't mind helping you out'. Amy jumped at the chance to get her PAD completed for other outstanding entries, she seemed pleased with Tony's response. (Observational fieldnotes taken whilst I was riding out on an ambulance in the West End of the city on 13/09/2014).

The implications of these practices on the veracity of academic standards, particularly in assessment practices, are significant and something which may be endemic throughout the students' clinical placements. Eaton (2019) found that:

> Whilst the ability to mentor paramedic students is a requirement of paramedic registration, unlike the national education requirements for teaching in higher education, there is no nationally accepted education process for practice educators to work within this role. Since the practice placements constitute approximately one-half of the paramedic

curriculum, it is surprising that there is no requirement for formal training or education of the clinicians who will support students during this
phase of their studies.

(Eaton, 2019: 1095)

McCall et al.'s (2009) and O'Meara's (2009) work found shortfalls in the
practice learning of paramedic students, suggesting a stronger partnership
between the university, ambulance service, and student is required to assure
the national quality and standards of clinical education. Students' epistemology formed within the structure of university education is not necessarily fully
transferred to the workplace. McCall et al. (2009) suggest that each party
needs to communicate and prepare for quality learning to occur. Arguably,
often ambulance service managers are more focused on meeting operational
demands and targets, than on student education, whilst students are usually
focused solely on the award of their degree, as Suchman et al. (2004) highlight in their work. These behaviours and practices can result in experienced
paramedics continuing their day-to-day working practices and procedures
which could be outdated, antiquated, obsolete, and at times fundamentally at
odds with the pedagogy and practice taught in the university setting, resulting in serious implications, not only in clinical placement pedagogy but also
in the assessment processes as well. We offer some recommendations later in
this chapter to help address these shortfalls.

Throughout my data collection, the notion of being an insider or outsider
researcher was at the forefront of my mind, as Brewer (2000) points out this
can have implications for the researcher's data. The next section of this chapter explores the relationship between my insider and outsider position as an
experienced paramedic/academic and as a researcher.

## 7.4 Insider-outsider researcher

The ethnography allowed me to really engage and witness firsthand how
and why students became so reliant on the subculture and hidden curriculum which O'Reilly (2009), Brewer (2000), Emerson et al. (2011), Walford
(2008), and Jeffrey (2014) also highlight in their work, claiming that ethnography can provide forms of in-depth data. It provided me with the opportunity to work with participants, to see and be part of their community of
practice (Lave & Wenger, 1991), and to share in their frustrations, anxieties,
disappointments, and at times sadness which confronted them in their challenging day-to-day work. The intricacies, nuances, colloquialisms, attitudes,
and behaviours become exposed, whilst I grappled with the emic position of
researcher as I became one of them (Brewer, 2000). I took Burgess's (1983)
advice, that the emic position provides the researcher with full participant
observation status who already belongs to the group being researched. At
the same time, I was reminded of Walford (2008) whose opinion highlights
the danger of the emic researcher going native as I was keen that my position

would not compromise my research findings. Considering the dichotomy between the emic and etic researcher and the potential influence on the study, we use this section of the chapter to illustrate how this dichotomy was managed in the field.

My insider observations helped guide me to slip between insider (emic) and outsider (etic) roles, to create a persona that encouraged and cajoled participants to disclose and illuminate more confidential and detailed accounts of their day-to-day practices. I was also aware that my research evolved through a reflexive stance related to my personal practice experience throughout the research. I took Hunt and Sampson's (2006) and van Maanen's (2011) advice to use reflexivity to examine the self and voice to help harness and understand the responsibility of the researcher within the research. I combined a meaningful personal, professional, and researcher self, to the research (van Maanen, 2011), as I became an integral part of the participants' community. I worked with them, and I copied their language, their slangy terms, their anecdotes, and at times their offensive language, to help cement my place within the community. Developments of social research, and in particular ethnography, have stimulated discussion on the advantages and disadvantages of 'insider' and 'outsider' researcher. For example, Allen (2004) believes:

> Advocates of the 'insider' view argue that it is only those who are closely immersed in the field of study who can ensure an authentic account. Others make the counterclaim, that the 'outsider' position is a preferable stance as it is free from the potential for bias that arises from too close an affiliation with the research subjects or 'going native'.
>
> (Allen, 2004: 15)

Burgess (1984) suggests situations are neither totally familiar nor totally strange, and the researcher's insider–outsider status changes at different points in a research project. I was also cognisant of O'Reilly's (2009) words that:

> The goal of ethnography, is to gain the perspective of the insider and to render it meaningful, raises special issues for ethnographers who are also members of the group they study.
>
> (O'Reilly, 2009: 109)

There were occasions, such as when I was required to treat patients as a paramedic, whereby I removed myself from the research process, then slipped back into the emic role as soon as I had cared for the patient (see Chapter 4). There were dichotomies within the discourse, as students releveled startling accounts of inappropriate behaviour, or I witnessed criminal damage to the ambulance (see Chapter 5). These actions often required me to switch between the emic and etic researcher as I continued with the ambulance shift. I questioned myself, at times, not really knowing what to do, whether to speak up or remain silent and ensure my acceptance into their workplace community. I provide two difficult and challenging examples here, which stretched and tested my professional and moral compass.

---

I was riding out with Rupert, a second year Foundation Degree student. This meant that Rupert was employed by the ambulance service as a student paramedic, who returned to university in blocks to commence his academic studies. This also meant that Rupert was working one-to-one with his crewmate (working partner), an experienced (old-timer) called Albert. The shift was due to start at 15–00 hours and finish at 23–00 hours at Newmoon ambulance station situated in the outskirts of the city. Albert arrived for the shift ten minutes late, although we had not received any emergency calls, so ambulance control was unaware of the situation. At 15–10 Albert arrived and parked his car on the station. I had not met the paramedic (Albert) before, but Rupert had been working with him for a whilst now and appeared to get on well with him. It was not long within the shift, after attending our second emergency call, that whilst sitting in the ambulance that I could smell alcohol on Albert's breath as we were talking. Albert was the driver of the ambulance that day and it soon became apparent that Albert had been drinking alcohol prior to starting the shift and driving the ambulance. I found a moment to speak with Rupert privately about my suspicions and to my surprise Rupert was aware of the situation, stating: 'Oh don't worry John (researcher) he often has a little drink before the shift, he only has a couple of pints at lunchtime, everyone knows him around here, it's okay it's just something he does'

Taken from my fieldnotes (12/12/2014).

---

On this occasion I was riding out with Jenny, a foundation degree student. Jenny was driving the ambulance whilst we had a patient in the back of the vehicle taking them to hospital. I sat in the front of the cab so I could talk to Jenny on route to hospital. The patient was in a stable condition, suffering just minor abdominal discomfort. Suddenly, jenny miscalculated the distance between a passing car and a parked motor vehicle (van) causing us to strike the parked van. I could see from looking through the ambulance wing mirror that we had shattered the van's

> right-hand side mirror, which was hanging from the vehicle with shattered glass and debris on the road as we continued passing various vehicles. I looked at Jenny who promptly said: 'pretend you didn't see that John (researcher)' and laughed as we continued on-route to hospital.
> Taken from my fieldnotes (06/08/2013).

The aforementioned two accounts taken from the fieldnotes go some way to illustrate the dichotomy of my insider/outsider relationship which had formed over time with the participants. O'Reilly (2009: 110) claims that it is the 'insiders' explicit goal to gain an insider perspective and to collect insider accounts'. It was therefore important for me to have their trust and assurance and be part of their community, if I were to witness and experience their real-life working relationships and behaviours. These were real and challenging dichotomies and ethical tensions which I had to grapple with as I spent time in the field as researcher.

In the next section of the chapter, we briefly reflect on my work and my experience as a researcher going into the research field to collect data. This section provides a summary of my feelings and experiences of the data collection within the field of ethnography.

## 7.5  Reflecting on the study

The title, 'An Examination of University Paramedic Students Enculturation into the Ambulance Service', was chosen for this research, firstly because of the unique opportunity we had to investigate what was really going on in the clinical practice setting and, secondly, it allowed me to witness the stagnant, sometimes hostile and difficult, practice environment which students can become exposed to.

When students spoke to me in my role as a university lecturer, rather than researcher, they often wanted to know why they were unable to demonstrate and disseminate the newly taught knowledge and skills formed within the university, into the workplace. They wanted to know why they had to work with experienced paramedics, who were often negative about teaching them and why these paramedics were opposed to university students. Furthermore, they asked me why I am giving up my time to be out with them 'on this wet and cold night shift?' (Jane, university student, 2014). I found myself unable to provide a satisfactory response, as I was left wondering and reflecting on my experiences as a novice ambulance man 40 years ago and asking myself why things had not fundamentally changed. This challenged my expectations as I confronted their reality.

As with any form of data collection, various strength and limitations emerge from the research process. In the next section, we highlight some of the strengths and limitations which this research offers.

## 7.6 Strengths and limitations of the study

Hammersley and Atkinson (2006) suggest the researcher makes these transparent within the narrative of the findings. In this section, we firstly highlight the strengths of this thesis before discussing some of the potential limitations of the research.

This research addresses a void within the literature on the paramedic student's enculturation into the working practice of the ambulance service. The data which we have collected over weeks and months of riding-out with student paramedics in the ambulance provides an insightful and meaningful account of the experiences of eight university paramedic students, along with many other consenting students and paramedics (participants), of whom I encountered whilst collecting data in the field. This work contributes to the body of knowledge around paramedic socialisation, as it depicts a paradox between the students' university studies and clinical workplace experience. These are important accounts which illustrate the fundamental premise of this book.

However, we acknowledge that there are some potential limitations of the study which need to be considered. For example, the convenience sample of participants became limited as participants volunteered to take part in the study. This meant that the selection process utilised purposeful sampling, as we had to rely on my own judgement when selecting participants to participate in the study, although one key purpose of this is to 'ensure that all criteria of relevance are included' (O'Reilly, 2009: 197). The nature of operational shift work also meant that I was restricted to who the participant (student) was crewed with (crewmate) on each shift. I was not able to impartially select who the student would be working with, as this was decided for me by the ambulance service rotas. Therefore, issues such as, ethnicity, gender, and age of participants were random. At times limited contact was made with the student's crewmate (paramedic) prior to arriving at the ambulance station to undertake the shift.

The data collection method, consisting of observations, fieldnotes, and interviews, became a lengthy and demanding process. This had the potential to impact on my intellectual resilience and physical stamina to record accurate data at times of tiredness and exhaustion. I managed this potential hazard by recognising my limitations, by having chocolate bars and sweets in my rucksack, along with a flask of coffee whilst in the field. This was particularly important whilst riding out on night shift after a day's work, as my resilience and personal stamina suffered in the early hours of the morning, especially on those shifts in the dark winter nights. I was also mindful of the possibility that participants, both students and experienced paramedics, may have acted in a style that favoured the researcher's expectations, along with my own prior experience and knowledge of the paramedic profession and NHS ambulance services, which Willis et al. (2010) suggest could be viewed as a limitation but also a strength. We suggest my knowledge and experience of the ambulance service and paramedic profession became a strength of this research. My insider perspective allowed me the opportunity to see the subtleties, nuances, and hidden aspects (Cresswell, 2009) of the workplace, which may not have been visible to outsider perspectives.

We believe that the reflective and reflexive approaches to the data collection, data analysis, interpretation, and representation of our findings, provided the checks and assurances, accountability, and honesty to this ethnographic account which Coffey and Atkinson (1996) and O'Reilly (2009) believe are the ethnographer's goals, as many of the findings from this research could confirm the transferability of findings to similar studies seen in peer-reviewed publications and reports associated with paramedic training and socialisation. Our rationale for choosing ethnography was, as O'Reilly (2011) suggests, to present a realistic representation that would assist in understanding the enculturation process, whilst also acknowledging the complexities of the socialisation process. As limited research exists on the enculturation of student paramedics, we drew on a qualitative research approach to provide a voice and offer a degree of insight into this area of research. Ethnography therefore provided an appropriate methodological lens for this study.

In the next section of this chapter, we offer some future direction and recommendations for policy and practice. We review the findings to offer potential solutions and recommendations which would add to the body of knowledge and contribute to practice.

## 7.7  Future directions and recommendations for policy and practice

The results drawn from our findings raise serious questions about some of the current practices carried out in the ambulance service. The future direction of paramedic development remains unclear and uncertain. Out-of-hospital emergency and urgent care continues to evolve and expand, whilst attrition of paramedics from the NHS ambulance service continues to be problematic and remains a priority for ambulance services to confront and address (ACCE, 2020). The retention of paramedics and the related recruitment problems are making retaining paramedics challenging.

We recognise that the research data was collected several years ago, although we would argue that potentially little has changed within the NHS ambulance service culture, attitudes, behaviours, or working practices. We provide several examples of paramedics fitness to practice hearings, taken from the HCPCS public website in 2023.

Case 1. You were convicted of making indecent photograph/pseudo-photograph of a child, namely 5 images of Category A, contrary to sections 1(1)(a) and 6 of the Protection of Children Act 1978.

Case 2. You were convicted on indictment of sexual assault on a male, which you did not inform the HCPC that you had been convicted of the offence outlined.

Case 3. You removed keys from the ignition of an ambulance and did not return those keys and/or disclose that you had taken them from ambulance when asked about their whereabouts by your employer.

Case 4. You tested positive for cannabis whilst at work at the Ambulance Response Service.

Case 5. You attended to patients and there were occasions when you did not:

a) undertake a detailed assessment and/or full patient history
b) recognise signs and symptoms in patients
c) recognise time critical patients
d) demonstrate the ability to act as lead clinician
e) treat patients appropriately

Case 6. You acted in an unprofessional and/or unsafe manner whilst driving an emergency vehicle in that:

a) on at least two occasions, you placed your mobile phone on the dashboard behind the vehicle's steering wheel and watched the playing video content.
b) on at least one occasion, you held your mobile phone handset to your left ear whilst on a call.
c) on at least one occasion, you held your mobile phone in your right hand and/or operated your mobile phone.

Case 7. You inappropriately demonstrated the use of your stethoscope on Colleague A, in that you moved the stethoscope onto Colleague A's left breast and pressed it on her left breast for approximately 10–30 seconds and you pushed your hands down the back of Colleague B's trousers, and/or grabbed the back of Colleague B's trousers and/or her underwear resulting in a 'wedgie'. You poked and/or smacked Colleague F on the back of the head and said 'come on fatty' or words to that effect. You said to Colleague F 'I would rather have my old crew member back as she was a good girl' or words to that effect. You said to Colleague F that 'I am going to punish you for your attitude by putting you over my knee and spanking you' or words to that effect.

We recognised that the aforementioned samples are a small percentage of the paramedic workforce, although we would liken these attitudes and behaviours with those depicted in our study several years ago. Therefore, we are not completely convinced that any significant change in behaviours, attitudes, or working practices has taken place since our initial research.

Our work is situated within social constructivism, as we draw on the work Lave and Wenger (1991) and Palincsar (1998) who looked at the social constructivist perspective on teaching, whilst Lave and Wenger (1991) situate learning as being socially constructed. They suggest that learning occurs in a social constructed environment such as the workplace. The environment influences and shapes the learning which occurs, such as that of the organisation (ambulance service), work colleagues in the environment (paramedics), and the various groups of practitioners who form bonds, such as those formed by paramedics in the watch-room or between students and paramedics. These all contribute to a form of learning, different from that which is taught in the university environment. Both these environments have different socially constructed ideas and assumptions, meaning the learning impacts on the student experience. This can hinder and curtail the type of pedagogy experienced in the workplace in the context of the informal workplace curriculum, as opposed to that formally prescribed in the university curriculum which can be significantly different. This poses pedagogical challenges for paramedic students (Devenish, 2014), as both the design and delivery of the formal curriculum fail to recognise and adequately address the real-life issues faced by paramedic students in the clinical workplace setting.

In the light of the aforementioned discussion, we are proposing that the information presented in this research may assist university paramedic students to better prepare for their clinical workplace. For example, it gives an indication of the processes which will confront paramedic students, such as the entrenched subculture which forms part of the student journey. This will provide students with a realistic expectation of the real-life working environment, rather than any perceived expectations drawn from media coverage or taken-for-granted assumptions. The research also highlights the various tensions which may exist between the university and ambulance cultures which identifies the processes of enculturation as students enter the paramedic workplace (Devenish, 2014) and the likely encounters they face as they transition into a registered paramedic. Newly qualified and experienced paramedics may also benefit from this research, as it identifies the subculture and subsequent hidden curriculum which results from it. As paramedics become mentors, this research provides a deeper and detailed insight into the student learning experience and how experienced paramedics might develop their mentoring styles and techniques to help support students, whilst dealing with the complexities of being expected to supervise new staff members. Furthermore, this research can be beneficial for paramedics as it identifies the forms of behaviour, storytelling, language, and identity, which fosters a deep-rooted cultural identity within the workplace.

Analytical propositions have been identified from this research, which informs the enculturation process encountered by university students. We provide our analytical propositions in the following, which we propose to address the concerns raised in this book.

1. A particular subculture exists within the ambulance service which students unexpectedly get drawn into as they attend their clinical practice placements. This subculture consists of forms of racism, homophobia, and sexist behaviours, along with criminal damage and cultural practices which are archaic and unacceptable in the current workplace environment. However, this appears ubiquitous and, to a degree, tolerated within the ambulance service, as the findings have depicted. To eradicate these archaic behaviours,

which are often targeted towards other staff members, students, and the public, we argue that a radical change to the current workplace culture is required. This would address the taken-for-granted, primitive, old-fashioned, and offensive practices evident in the ambulance service, if the paramedic profession is to strive for professional status. The findings suggest that resilience to these challenging and unacceptable behaviours was not sufficiently addressed in the undergraduate paramedic curriculum. University paramedic programmes should question the need to invite ambulance service representatives to attend and address the university programme ensuring content reflects the reality of the practice placement setting. Empowering educators of ambulance trusts to actively promote equality, diversity, and inclusion, through clear expectations of behaviour, would go some way to address these concerns. Students deserve to feel safe and secure when attending clinical placements, and to be able to challenge and report unacceptable behaviours when they occur, which currently is not necessarily the case.

2. The findings indicate that a patchwork of standards exists regarding paramedic mentorship and Practice Placement Educators (PPEDs). The role and responsibilities of qualified paramedic practitioners are of concern. The public expect a speedy response when they require the services of the paramedic. They deserve a kind, reassuring, knowledgeable, and skilful practitioner to attend to them who has been assessed to the highest standard, who can confidently and competently address the patients presenting clinical complaint and concerns. Patients are often in their greatest need, the most vulnerable in society, those who have suffered significant physical injury or complex physical illness along with mental health issues, people who are at their lowest ebb, and people who just need help. However, our findings reveal that the current model of mentorship training may not provide this assurance (Givati et al., 2018), as obsolete, outdated, and inconsistent standards of mentorship training and education appear common throughout the findings. Some ambulance services, however, fully engage with universities who offer postgraduate studies in mentorship-related subjects, whilst other ambulance services offer their staff a one- or two-day in-house (ambulance service) mentorship training course, although some ambulance services have no formal structure and expect paramedics to take on the role of mentor, as highlighted by Eaton (2019). The diverse forms of mentorship education and training are considerably different, both in their expectations, knowledge, and standards. This approach to paramedic mentorship is broken and does not work. It is inconsistent, erratic, conflicting, and inconceivable in today's modern NHS ambulance service.

The findings indicate that there is a strong case for an agreed nationally recognised paramedic mentorship programme, similar to those of the Nursing and Midwifery Council (NMC, 2028) and the Department of Education's Academic Mentor Programme (National Association of School-Based Teacher Trainers, 2020), to bring paramedic mentorship in line with similar professional organisations.

3. The final recommendation arising from this research relates to the existing paramedic workforce, who qualified prior to the introduction of

paramedic degree-level qualifications. Although limited now in numbers, these experienced paramedics, often referred to throughout the findings as 'old-timers' (Lave & Wenger, 1991), require clinical updates and continuous professional development (CPD) in areas such as patient assessment and management, ethics and law, and behavioural studies. Further development and training would ensure this group of practitioners become and remain current and knowledgeable in the educational developments occurring within the profession as taught to student paramedics at university. As our data suggests, many experienced paramedics (old-timers), felt isolated from the current knowledge afforded to the new cadre of students and newly graduated paramedics. This development could be carried out over several weeks and months through a university development programme.

## 7.8 Conclusion

Our work offers unique insight into the day-to-day realities of traditional working practices to which student paramedics become exposed. Devenish's (2014) work helps to illustrate this by exploring the transition from being a university student to becoming a practising intern paramedic in Australia through the lens of existing professional socialisation theories. Schein (2004) provides a framework to help us understand the three distinguishable components of organisational culture, whilst Lave and Wenger's (1991) theoretical model of communities of practice gives substance and theoretical underpinning to this work. The paramedic student journey is an unsettled and often uneven pathway which students are expected to navigate, often under challenging and difficult conditions, at times with little, if any, support or encouragement. Therefore, this research is a timely contribution to the limited literature on the enculturation of the UK paramedic students, as they go from university into the workplace.

The research has considered the expectations of student paramedics as they become exposed to the unexpected reality of the workplace. The formal and informal models of curriculum have been discussed, and issues around subculture, and marginalisation, have been alluded to when discussing this research. Notwithstanding this, we believe these results will contribute to the overall body of knowledge on the enculturation of student paramedics' curriculum development and policy and practice with regard to the UK NHS ambulance service and paramedic profession. Finally, the experiences of the participants within this study offer a rich and detailed ethnographic insight into the ambulance service for individuals wishing to pursue a career in the paramedic profession. We refer to the work of Givati et al. (2018) to conclude this book.

> Over the past two decades, paramedic education has undergone a process of academisation and a shift from in-house, occupational training to university-based undergraduate programmes. While the professional regulation and standardisation of Allied Health Professionals' education has captured scholarly attention, the study of paramedic practice is still in

its infancy and there is a need to explore its evolvement in relation to the fluid societal–political circumstances affecting its provision and demand.

(Givati et al., 2018: 353)

The illustration in Figure 7.1 provides an overview of the student paramedic journey as we see it, as they go from student (novice) through to becoming registered healthcare professionals (expert). We illustrate the various stages which students go through, whilst highlighting some of the influencing factors which impact on these. Connecting arrows link the student journey whilst the broken (dotted) line captures the whole journey, incorporating students' legitimate peripheral participation through to full legitimate participation into the community of practice (Lave & Wenger, 1991).

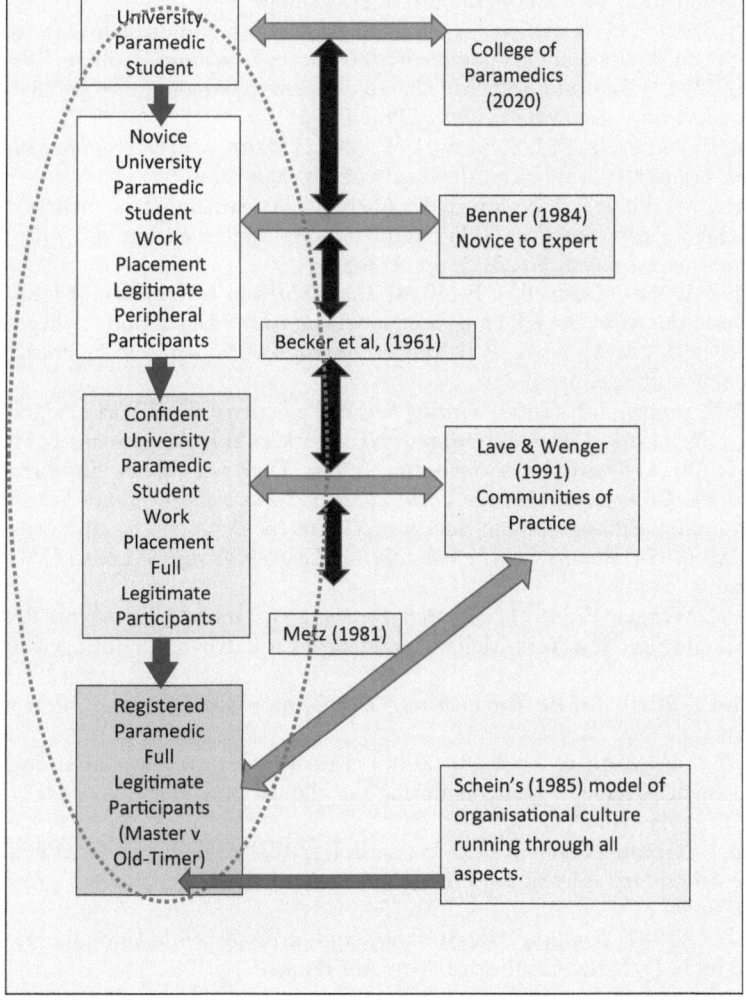

*Figure 7.1* The student journey.

## References

Allen, D. (2004) 'Ethnomethodological insight into insider-outsider relationships in nursing ethnographies of healthcare settings', *Nursing Inquiry*, 11(1), pp. 14–24.

Association of Ambulance Chief Executives (AACE). (2020) https://aace.org.uk/

Boychuck Duchscher, J. E. (2009) 'Transition shock: The initial stage of role adaptation for newly graduated registered nurses', *Journal of Advanced Nursing*, 65(5), pp. 1103–1113.

Brewer, J. D. (2000) *Ethnography: Understanding Social Research*. Buckingham/ Philadelphia, PA: Open University Press.

Burgess, R. G. (1983) *In the Field*. London: Allen & Unwin.

Coffey, A. & Atkinson, P. (1996) *Concepts and Coding. Making Sense of Qualitative Data: Complementary Research Strategies*. Thousand Oaks/London/New Delhi: SAGE Publishing, pp. 26–53.

Cresswell, J. W. (2009) *Research Design, Qualitative, Quantitative and Mixed Methods Approaches*, 3rd ed. London: SAGE Publishing.

Devenish, A. S. (2014) 'Experiences in becoming a paramedic: A qualitative study examining the university qualified paramedics', *Creative Education*, 7(6), pp. 786–801.

Eaton, G. (2019) 'Learning values in shared decision-making in undergraduate paramedic education', *Journal in Clinical Practice*, 25.

Emerson, R. M., Fretz, R. I. & Shaw, L. L. (2011) *Writing Ethnographic Fieldnotes*, 2nd ed. London/Chicago: The University of Chicago Press.

Givati, A., Markham, C. & Street, K. (2018) 'The bargaining of professionalism in emergency care practice: NHS paramedics and higher education', *Advances in Health Science Education*, 23(2), pp. 353–369.

Hafferty, F. W. & O'Donnell, J. F. (2014) *The Hidden in Curriculum in Health Professional Education*, 1st ed. Hanover, New Hampshire: Dartmouth College Press.

Hammersley, M. & Atkinson, P. (2006) *Ethnography: Principles in Practice*, 3rd ed. London: Routledge, pp. 1–3.

Hunt, C. & Sampson, F. (2006) *Writing Self & Reflexivity*. New York: Palgrave.

Jackson, P. W. (1968) *Life in Classrooms*. New York, NY: Holt, Reinhart & Winston.

Jeffrey, B. (2014) *The Primary School in Testing Times: A Classic Ethnography of a Creative, Community Engaged, Entrepreneurial and Performance School*. New York/London: Ethnography in Education Conference.

Kramer, M. (1974) *Reality Shock: Why Nurses Leave Nursing*. St Louis: C.V. Mosby Company.

Lave, J. & Wenger, E. (1991) *Situated Learning: Legitimate Peripheral Participation*. Cambridge/New York/Melbourne/Madrid/Cape Town: Cambridge University Press.

'Look east'. (2020) *British Broadcasting Corporation (BBC) News*, 30 September 2020.

McCall, L., Wray, N. & Lord, B. (2009) 'Factors affecting the education of pre-employment paramedic students during the clinical practicum', *Journal of Emergency Primary Health Care*, 7(4).

McCann, L., Granter, E., Hyde, P. & Hassard, J. (2013) 'Still blue-collar after all these years? An ethnography of the professionalisation of emergency work', *Journal of Management Studies*, 50(5), pp. 750–774.

Metz, L. D. (1981) *Running Hot-Structure and Stress in Ambulance Work*, 1st ed. Edited by L. D. Metz. Cambridge, MA: Abt Books.

National Association of School-Based Teacher Trainers. (2020) https://www.nasbtt. org.uk/#:~:text=Welcome%20to%20The%20National%20Association,imple mentation%20of%20national%20policy%20developments

Nursing and Midwifery Council. (2008) https://www.nmc.org.uk/globalassets/site documents/standards/nmc-standards-to-support-learning-assessment.pdf

O'Meara, P. (2009) 'Professional and community expectations of rural ambulance services in Australia, pp2', *The Australian Journal of Paramedicine*, 1(3–4), pp. 1–7.

O'Reilly, K. (2009) *Key Concepts in Ethnography*. London: SAGE Publishing.

O'Reilly, K. (2011) *Ethnographic Methods*, 2nd ed. London/New York: Routledge.

Palincsar, A. S. (1998) 'Social constructivist perspectives on teaching and learning', *Annual Review of Psychology*, 49, 345–375.

Reynolds, L. (2004) 'Is prehospital care really a profession', *Journal of Emergency Primary Health Care*, 2.

Schein, H. E. (2004) *Organizational Culture and Leadership*, 3rd ed. San Francisco. CA: Jossey- Bay.

Suchman, L. A., Williamson, R. P., Litzelman, K. D., Frankel, M. R., Mossbarger, L. D., Inui, S. T. & The Relationship-Centred C. I. D. T. (2004) 'Towards an informal curriculum that teaches professionalism-transforming the social environment of a medical school', *General Internal Medicine*, 19, pp. 501–504.

van Maanen, J. (2011) *Tales of the Field: On Writing Ethnography*, 2nd ed. Chicago/ London: The University of Chicago.

Walford, G. (2008) *How to do Educational Ethnography*. London: Tufness Press.

Wankhade, P. & Mackway-Jones, K. (2015) *Understanding the Management of Ambulance Services Ambulance Services: Leadership and Management Perspectives*. Cham/Heidelberg/New York/Dordrecht/London: Springer.

Willis, E., Williams, B., Brightwell, R., O'Meara, P. & Pointon, T. (2010) 'Road-ready paramedics and the supporting sciences curriculum', *Focus on Health Professional Education: A Multi-Disciplinary Journal*, 11(2), pp. 1–13.

# Index

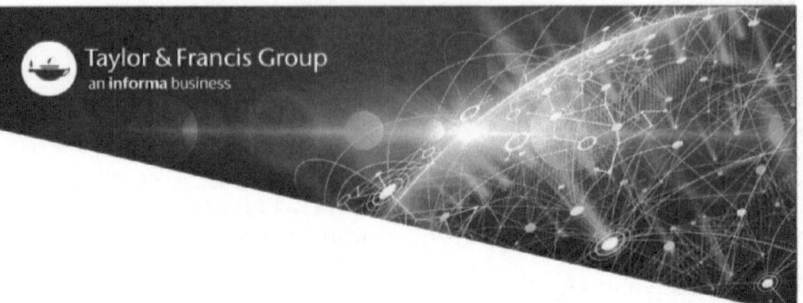
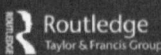
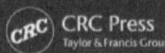